The DOCTOR
and the
STORK

THE DOCTOR AND THE STORK

A MEMOIR OF
MODERN MEDICAL BABYMAKING

K.K. GOLDBERG

SHE WRITES PRESS

Published 2015
Printed in the United States of America
ISBN: 978-1-63152-830-9
Library of Congress Control Number: 2015942224

Design by Stacey Aaronson

For information, address:
She Writes Press
1563 Solano Ave #546
Berkeley, CA 94707

She Writes Press is a division of SparkPoint Studio, LLC.

For Kenneth

Author's Note

Though one in thirty babies born in the United States is a twin, when I became pregnant with twins at the tender age of thirty-nine, I couldn't find a book that mirrored my experience. There were wonderful titles that offered medical expertise, nutritional advice, and occasionally strategies for self-care, but nothing that spoke honestly about mental survival for the mother—the emotional aspects of gestating two. Though every twin pregnancy is unique, the one common factor is that it's a whole different ball game than carrying a single baby.

If you are pregnant with twins, or pregnant after a struggle with infertility, I hope that my story will amuse, comfort, distract, and accompany you on your journey. If you are reading this for other reasons, I hope the same. In case it needs saying, none of this book should be construed as medical advice. A doctor's word on your situation is the only one that counts.

While this memoir explores the ambivalence, angst, and discomfort that can come with a post-IVF twin pregnancy, I'd like to say up front that I consider twins a blessing beyond compare. Hindsight offers a view less blurred by hormones, uncertainty, and fear.

I can see, looking back, how lucky I have been. Many women go through far greater hardships, with far greater grace. I'm grateful every day for the gifts I've been given, for my friends, for this family, even for the struggles of the pregnancy itself, the rigors of which kicked my butt and opened my heart.

WEEK ONE:

IVF IS the EXtReme SPORt Of InfeRtiLitY

Here's something I learned about infertility: what's hard is all that *doesn't* happen, the sameness and the wait. It was one more birthday grinding past, the odds darker with each candle I blew out. It was the aunt who said every spring, "Happy Mother's Day—even though you're not a mother." It was our social circle begetting like the Bible, and crying when my old friend shared her happy news. That's when I knew it wasn't only my ovaries that were in trouble. Before infertility, I'd always thought of suffering as tolerating loss, accepting change. Three years into it, I understood that lack of change could ache just as much.

Maybe that was why when Ken and I headed to the FedEx store to pick up our box of drugs, $5,000 worth, shipped overnight, I felt so incredibly tired, despite having slept twelve hours the night before. As much as I dreaded IVF, as many times as I had said, "That's not for me," here we were, counting the hours until the first shot.

I told myself at least it was something to *do*, something besides waiting. By then I spoke acronym—I knew the difference between FSH (mine was high) and HSG (tubes were open)—and had done an MRI, along with two saline sonograms and a fibroid surgery. I'd rejected IUI, so all that remained now was IVF. It was the extreme sport of the fertility world, in terms of pain and cost, but I'd turned thirty-nine and my husband, Ken, was forty-two. We'd been snowed in at base camp after years of training. It was time to make the climb.

So I balanced the package beneath my chin, arms held straight at my hips. It wasn't heavy, at least not in the literal sense. I felt mild surprise, upon seeing it, that this carton, filled with needles, vials, suppositories, pills, and a red plastic sharps container, had my name on it. With that freight, there was no turning back. I should mention that I distrusted doctors and feared almost everything related to traditional medicine. For me, these drugs were potions from a voodoo priest. They seemed to work for some people, though—about one in four.

It was a sunny Saturday in Berkeley. We'd driven to FedEx directly from puppy school, with Friso, a four-month-old bichon, curled on my lap. He looked part piglet and part lamb, and he panted with contentment—the precise opposite of my emotional state.

"I think we learned more in puppy class today than Friso did," I said, after settling our cargo into the trunk, neither of us talking about the parcel. Another thing I'd learned about infertility: it didn't really help to talk about it.

"We learned that our puppy thinks 'sit' means 'zoom in a giant circle,'" Ken said.

"We could easily end up with a TUD"—our code for "totally untrained dog." I hugged Friso. He licked my face.

At home, we unloaded our pharmaceutical trove onto the dining room table, and Ken penciled out a careful inventory: Menopur, Ganirelix, Endometrin, HCG, doxycycline, names like ancient gods, to be chanted in low tones.

"The Follistim needs to be refrigerated," Ken said.

"Like a cool summer wine," I joked. I didn't need to cry. My tear ducts, like my ovaries, were wearing out. Besides, it upset Friso. I scooped up the Follistim and stacked the six zippered packets in the deli drawer, with the garlic hummus and jack cheese.

The rest of the medication could sit in the room we'd once casually called "the nursery," then "the empty room," then, in desperation, "the nap room," and finally "the second bedroom." We put the box beneath the windows that looked out on the yard and the oak. Standing side by side, we stared.

This altar of cardboard contained not just our possible future, but also all that had led us to this point, the trail littered with ovulation kits, basal thermometers, Clomid bottles, and pregnancy strips with only one line. Our third Christmas of infertility, after the fibroid surgery and right before our birthdays, the lights and the gatherings and the gifts had tipped me into feelings of doom. Once again, nothing particular had happened—just the noticeable passing of time, the particular battery of holidays. After New Year's, I had considered joining an infertility support group, hideous as that sounded, and talked to the discussion leader by phone. I'd cringed at the background noises, her cooing infant daughter, apparently the product of IVF. When I stopped semihating the woman, I wondered, for the first time, why I shouldn't cross this final line. How much worse could IVF be than a support group?

"You're old," the doctor at the fertility clinic had told me at our first meeting. "Your eggs are old." Of course, she hadn't said it like that—those facts were coded in talk of follicles and supply. Actually what she'd said was, "People suffering from infertility have higher rates of depression and anxiety than those with cancer."

The onslaught of treatment would be intense. I woke nights dry-mouthed and quivery at the thought of the shots, the hormones, the ultrasounds and blood draws, but mostly I feared it would all come to nothing. Ken, a scientist, understood the statistical spread on IVF, how the slant of success cratered with age. For me those numbers towered, an avalanche that could crush our dream.

Now, as we stood before the box, the rumble of the odds grew silent. IVF was a gesture. Finally, we would show the gods we were serious about children. Despite having spent tens of thousands of dollars to reach this medical moment, I still held most important those forces beyond science— faith, luck, and the magic of belief itself.

"I'm kind of excited," Ken said, as if reading my mind.

"Me, too," I admitted, and a strange spark lit my fatigue.

There was power that came in defying my own dread. After all, I'd met Ken through JDate, another thing I'd said I'd never do. Our paths would never have crossed anywhere but cyberspace, so maybe our DNA also needed technology to meet. We'd be a modern family in every way. If we could fall in love online, just maybe we could make a baby in a dish.

I stashed a bottle of Ambien in a bedside drawer. I'd asked our doctor to throw this in so I wouldn't lie awake at night, hopped up on hormones and haunted by poor percentages. I wanted to avoid that one most dangerous drug, no matter its short-term lift: hope. I'd been dealing with the side effects of hope for years. It's not the final ascent to the peak that's hard. It's the journey back down where the hazards accrue. Still, I believed if only I could get pregnant, the long wait would end.

AS THE FIRST INJECTION LOOMED, I trusted Ken could remember what we had covered in our "orientation"—six of us at the clinic, crammed into a windowless room, under the watchful eye of our assigned nurse. There, we had practiced loading needles from vials and injecting three-inch cubes of fake fat, each square of flesh-colored Jell-O smudged from so much handling.

It was weird to be with other couples. Our friends had stopped inviting us to their kids' first and second birthdays —granting a perimeter of privacy that felt a lot like loneliness. Infertility had been so isolating, so secret and obvious both. Now, suddenly, we had a small dinner party of relatable people. For something that felt so solitary, this not-happening happened to a lot of us.

One woman, who had done the injections before, gave us tips. She had wielded the syringe herself, she announced; her husband couldn't. Next to her, hip in a leather jacket and black cap, he grinned sheepishly.

"Use ice each time," she said. "Pinch the chunk of skin

you inject." The pain of the pinch distracted from the pain of the poke. It was brilliant.

At one point, fiddling with the plunger on the practice syringe, I accidentally squirted water across the table, into her husband's eye. Everyone laughed while I apologized profusely. For a moment, it was all a festive science project.

Then, out of the blue, the other woman mentioned her first child. Earlier, the nurse had warned us not to pick up heavy things. "Is it okay if I lift my daughter? She weighs thirty pounds."

I suppressed a loud sigh. I felt as if she said this to distinguish herself from the rest of us, those who couldn't do what she had done. Why was she there? I wondered. Who needed more than one child? One child had always been our plan, then our prayer, and now our desperate bid. I crossed my arms. I didn't look at her until the end, when she touched my elbow and said, "Good luck" in a trembling voice.

"Good luck, too," I said, my voice also raw, meaning it despite my petty self.

Now, we'd arrived at cycle day one—the place we returned to month after month. I stretched, laced up my shoes, and went for a long, final run. There would be no vigorous exercise allowed through IVF. *God, and Ganirelix, please help us. We only want one.*

BY THE END OF WEEK ONE, we were halfway through the IVF shots and halfway through the TV series *Lost*—four seasons' worth rented on DVD. I couldn't fully escape myself, but it helped to watch a planeload of buff people marooned on an island as Ken and I huddled on an island of our own, the chocolate-stained couch in the office–man cave–TV room.

IVF, like infertility, turned me inward. Barely anyone knew we'd taken the plunge. I dreaded being asked, "Did it work?" The questions hurt. There were still the people who blithely inquired, "So, do you guys want to have kids?" One family friend liked to wink at me and whisper, "You have a bun in the oven?" Perhaps I looked progressively fatter. Even worse were the few who'd been clued in and needed updates, as if we could make slow progress on infertility, like building a chair: *we've got the legs; shaping the arms now.* Of course, the lowest life form was people who offered tips, like "stop eating tofu," or "just try to relax." Faking okayness took too much work and was only slightly less awful than honesty.

I'd been able to talk to my old friend Tina, who had suffered through three miscarriages. Then she'd gone and gotten pregnant—with twins—and, in a numbness of envy, in the selfishness that comes with feeling victimized, I hadn't done much more than click "like" on the Facebook photos of her tremendous form. I felt left behind, and ashamed that I couldn't rise to the occasion. I wanted only one baby, but the thought of two, all at once—the bounty seemed immense.

My friend Linda, who was childfree by choice, also knew we'd started IVF. Instead of offering advice, she brought brown rice and green veggies, took Friso around the block. Her words were among the few that helped. "Whatever happens, it's going to be the right thing," she would say. "When you look back, you'll be able to see that."

Now, there wasn't much to look back on yet, but we could look steadily at the TV. *Lost* took us from dinner to injections, that particularly difficult segment of waiting.

Each night at nine o'clock, Ken returned to the dining room to load up the Menopur and Follistim, poring over notes and murmuring at each syringe, "There's a reason I became a physicist and not a medical doctor."

The child of a doctor and a nurse, Ken hated the sight of blood, couldn't stand needles. Above all, he hated being helpless about my hurt. "I would do this if I could," he said, meaning bear the baby. I believed him. Ken shied away from hyperbole, except when driving, when he liked to scream at the pokey Priuses of Berkeley, "You have no will to live!" Otherwise he was the calmest person I knew, and patient. Days at the lab, he studied nanodots on glass (though he couldn't find larger items at home, like his shoes, socks, keys, and wallet). He loved animals and with stubborn integrity had refused to eat them since age four. Bald and bearded, he was a guys' guy, with his baseball and T-shirts and gadgets, but he had a tender side. Based on something I'd told him about my girlhood, he'd cased the city of Baltimore, while there to give a talk, to get me unicorn stickers. Early in our dating, I knew I could have kids with him.

At ten o'clock, we met in the bedroom, needles arrayed on a plate, set carefully on top of Friso's crate. The puppy's snores formed the backdrop to our choked-up conversation.

"This medicine is helping us," I said, wanting a positive spin.

"Did you do the ice?" Ken's hands shook as he held the first needle.

"Yes, I'm numb."

"Should we do the pinching thing?"

"Jam it in. Seriously. Let's be done."

Ken's eyes grew watery, and he gripped each syringe in a fist, using his thumb to depress the plunger. When it was done, I praised his technique.

"You're totally lying."

"It was better than last night."

In that week alone, I'd had more shots than in the last thirty years combined, as a former avoider of all things medical. To top it off, I downed Ambien like hard candy. It brought sleep like a tide rising, and, before popping in orange foam earplugs and topping off with Advil, I whispered out an overdose of hope.

"We are going to have a family," I said.

Our foreheads touched. Ken spoke softly, too. "We're a family already," he said.

Here's something else I learned about infertility: you test the fibers of your bonds, the ropes that hold you on the mountain's steepest slope when your own footing fails. In the midst of all that waiting, in the dizzy dangling of uncertainty, I knew his words were true.

I dreamed of two blimps cruising over an ocean break, then plunging into the water, where they turned to submarines.

WEEK TWO:

The TWIN PARADOX

By cycle day eight of IVF—which is how you mark time through infertility treatment—my abdomen turned puffy, bruised, and sore. As we drove to our "preop" visit at the clinic, the waistband of my jeans, the pressure of the seat belt, ached against my swollen organs. The hormones had pushed my follicles to turn up fourteen eggs. I felt like an Easter basket, overflowing with fragile cargo, fragile feelings.

We faced Dr. Marion across a desk. Though it was early on a Saturday, she wore a white lab jacket over a skirt, stockings, and heels and talked to us in her standard verbal dash, as if someone had slipped a pinch of cocaine into her coffee. That she spoke one notch more slowly than an auctioneer made her seem smart and devoted to beating even the most urgently ticking biological clock. We'd waited three years to have a baby—why let another hour fritter away? She had a runner's build, speed in all things, and she'd get us pregnant fast.

"From that bruised melon belly of yours, we'll probably

get eight good eggs, and with some luck, after fertilization, the Darwinian rat race will leave you with about five ass-kicking blastocysts."

Of course she didn't say those words exactly, but she did mention "five blasts." It sounded like a party, or an explosion.

"How do you feel about multiples?" she asked, leaning back to study us.

"Multiples?" I didn't understand the word in this context, though it would soon come to define my life.

"Twins or triplets."

Of course, I knew twins often came from IVF, but I figured that happened to Brad and Angelina, or J. Lo, people who didn't have to stand in line at airports or worry about co-pays. Then there was my friend Tina in Vermont, who'd come by her twins naturally. She made her own maple syrup, was handy with an ax, could run in snowshoes. She taught science to eighth graders. That was the other kind of person who could handle "multiples."

I loved to nap in the afternoon, read novels at night. Despite all the resting, I rarely felt relaxed or mellow. When Friso rejected his kibble, I'd fret for hours, churn out questions to a bichon chat board. When Friso threw up, I called Ken at work.

"Is it chunky or just bile?" he would ask in a quiet voice.

"It's yellow, and smooth."

"Hang on, I'll step out of my meeting." Ken wasn't laid-back either.

Once, as Friso suffered an episode of spastic gasping, we raced him to the vet, who diagnosed "a sneeze."

So when Dr. Marion asked us about having multiples,

Ken and I locked eyes. Our plan had always been *one*. One baby I could haul to Peet's Coffee, tote on my hip. One baby could be handed off to Ken or handed back to me. We could pour all our love and concern into one vessel, give him or her the best. Our house had one extra bedroom. Where would we put a second child? In the man cave, with the burrito wrappers and TV?

With one baby, I wouldn't come close to the constellation of my family of origin and would thereby keep us safe from chaos and collapse. I'd come from a two parent–two child nuclear family, and we'd imploded in the great shock wave of 1970s divorce. The radioactive decay still plumed around us decades later. A triad, plus puppy, seemed far more stable. All these factors hovered in my pause.

"Twins would be a miracle," I said at last. "We have enough love for twins."

My head jerked to Ken as if I'd just suffered hormonally induced Tourette's. He looked as surprised as I to hear these words from my mouth, this speaking in tongues. The last time I had used the word "miracle" was in relation to a never-ending tube of toothpaste. I had specifically avoided the term in discussions of fertility. I even disliked the word "fertile," which seemed vaguely flaky and also designed to make you feel you would not, in fact, be able to have children.

Now, a distant part of my mind shrilled a protest: *The plan is one! One husband, one puppy, one baby!* Still, something stopped me from contradicting what I'd said aloud. Here's another thing I learned during IVF: your head, heart, and body may have competing dreams.

Meanwhile, Ken nodded. I wasn't sure if he acquiesced

or thought the decision was mine. He'd always wanted a handful of kids, though he agreed with me on what was best: just one.

Dr. Marion responded, "If you have twins, your life, like your body, will be stretched to the limit. If you have triplets, you're fucked." Of course, what she really said was, "The pregnancy could be more difficult, complications more likely. There are higher percentages of miscarriage, prematurity, birth defects."

"I would worry about that stuff with one," I shrugged. In truth, I'd barely given pregnancy a thought. It seemed like the finish line, not the beginning, a blip on the reproductive timeline. Nine months of eating Coconut Bliss ice cream and doing prenatal yoga seemed like nothing next to three years of infertility—practically a vacation. I'd always been athletic, and figured carrying a baby would be another kind of workout. I would run a bit slower, walk Friso at half pace.

"For your size, you could just handle twins. What are you, five four?"

"Five three and a half," I clarified. Ken and I suppressed chuckles that usually came with this topic—he claimed I had added an inch on JDate. Now it was medically relevant.

"Three percent of couples in your position get triplets. That would be considered extremely high risk for you."

"Triplets would be a hardship," I agreed. "I don't want my own reality show."

Dr. Marion didn't smile. She likely didn't know who Snooki was, or who would be the next Bachelorette. Infertility had acquainted us with the lowest rungs of TV, though

IVF had given me a sense of permission, a sense of mercy toward myself, that I'd long misplaced. I now believed in doing whatever made everything else easier, even if that meant reruns of *The Millionaire Matchmaker*.

"We don't want to be outnumbered," I explained. "We have a puppy."

"Our goal is always single pregnancies," she affirmed.

Dr. Marion gave us a densely printed form, which reminded me of the "handouts" I used to distribute as an English teacher in community college. *You will be tested—you can't say you weren't warned.*

"We ask you to sign this, though of course it isn't binding." The page said we understood the "risk" of multiples. There were boxes to check about what we'd do with triplets: go with the risky birth or opt for "reduction." The word left me blank, then surprised, then sad. I understood that IVF might succeed or might fail, but an unintended third course—that, I could not grasp.

Besides, handing us the idea of pregnancy halfway through IVF was like tossing rope to climbers stranded in an icy crevasse and warning them with a shout, "This may chafe your palms!" If anything, I delighted in Dr. Marion's belief that we could have a baby at all. Another doctor had rated my chances of conception at 1 percent. My acupuncturist had been mentioning "all the kids already out there who need loving homes."

The thought of "reduction," of willfully ending a life we'd fought to create, was painful even to consider, but neither of us imagined it would come to pass. The point of the "nonbinding" form was to force us to squint at the fine print and thereby stave off precisely the denial I now eagerly embraced. Multiple babies seemed a little like the side effects they speed-speak at the end of every drug commercial. *May cause racing heart sleep eating sudden death uncontrolled diarrhea.* You never think you will be the one.

We had enough love for twins. But enough time, money, skill? An eight-pound bichon ruled our household. We weren't exactly naturals. Still, the thought of twins gave me a pang. I couldn't deny the magic of two, as if they could choose, as if they'd come as a pair.

After three minutes of hushed chat, curt nods, and stilted "uh-huhs," we checked off that we'd be okay with twins. For triplets, we marked "reduction." The notion tunneled my vision with gray. I knew I couldn't carry three, but that gesture of the pen sharpened the grief I'd been carrying with infertility, pinpointing one more way in which I was prefailing—at even the earliest and most hypothetical levels of parenthood. A different woman would have said *never.* For all the clinical precision IVF brings to conception, for all its gifts, there's an equal and opposite terror, a burden that comes with bypassing nature. At the same time we were strangely rushed, a little shamefaced, and too casual, as if not discussing life and death but weighing an expensive cup-holder option on a new car. I felt queasy as we passed the paper back.

Three percent of IVFers ended up with three fetuses. IVF worked for only one in four people, and of those, about 20 percent ended up with twins. I couldn't do all the math but decided there was no reason to think our first round of IVF would work on overdrive.

In Einstein's physics, the "twin paradox" is a thought

experiment in which one twin orbits the earth at near light speed, then returns to find his brother an old man. In IVF, the twin paradox is the fact that transferring two embryos ups your chance for one baby, sometimes by as much as 10 percent, and if you finish the cycle without getting pregnant at all, you will, without a doubt, have aged. You'll return to Infertilityville, out $12,000, ovaries tired, heart smashed.

On the car ride home, I said again to Ken, "We really want just one, right?"

"Yeah," he said.

"That's the plan," I said, so the gods would hear us, too, update our request. Later it would seem they did, and laughed.

Week Three:

It Takes a Village to Make a Child (or Two)

In the empty waiting room of the clinic, the scent of fresh coffee filled the air, a reminder of my old life, when I'd wake up and savor a cup of Guatemalan, rather than pounding a quart of water to enlarge my bladder for a medical procedure. It was 6:00 a.m. on our "transfer day," and Ken and I had the foyer to ourselves. I hunkered down to watch an episode of *30 Rock* on my iPad.

I knew I could be praying or meditating, but at the moment Tina Fey seemed better than religion. The Valium I'd taken on the car ride had left me loose and calm, a sensation limited by my abdominal organs, which felt packed together like wobbling water balloons. Someone had set stale-looking bagels beneath a banner that read WE PARTICIPATE IN NATIONAL INFERTILITY AWARENESS DAY, as if it were a celebratory occasion.

A nurse I'd never seen before summoned us from the lobby, and for once they didn't weigh me or measure me to make sure I was still five foot three–ish and 115 pounds.

We followed her down the hallway, through a thick door, to a windowless space, where a man in a suit leaned over a desk to chat with two uniformed nurses, as if at a bar. She led me past the curtained hutch with a cot where, five days before, I'd awaited my egg retrieval surgery. While it is considered the most "invasive" part of IVF—and requires general anesthesia—it also seemed like a welcome break. For the last year I'd been wide awake while doctors and techs performed prison-level body searches for the purpose of diagnoses. It seemed better to "sleep" through the needle that would be threaded into my ovaries, so for once I'd climbed up on the table with minimal sogginess at the eyes. Just before the oxygen cup descended over my mouth, I'd chatted with the masked doctor about my recent piece in the *New York Times*, feeling like God would not let me die here after throwing me such a major bone.

The procedure had yielded twelve eggs, a perfect dozen. Of those, seven had been fertilized.

Now, the next big event had arrived. We stepped through a door on the left into the transfer room.

Maybe it was the Valium, but for the first time since I had begun IVF, I felt awed by the process. We were so close to where the embryos were stored, to the secret forces of fate and biology that could turn those little cocktails of human DNA into breathing babies.

Behind a second door, marked LAB, our 120-micron whippersnappers were enjoying the most expensive day care they would ever experience. Last we'd heard, we had five good "blasts," as Dr. Marion had predicted.

Ken helped me up onto the chair, a more daunting

platform than usual, with the foot hooks at a crazy angle.

"Yikes," I whispered.

It looked more like a contraption for giving birth, with your legs splayed like a turkey for the roast. Luckily, the Valium, and my sense of homestretch anticipation, kept me from spiraling into a further fit of resistance. Through the haze and discomfort, I even felt a tickle of excitement. I wanted to hear about how our DNA was faring, if the Team Goldberg Cellular League would be going to the finals. How many of our blasts had been benched, and how many would play? Minutes away from the transfer, we still did not know.

Every day since the big harvest, we had waited nervously for Dr. Marion's evening phone updates on our embryos. Each time, some got cut. Others seemed sturdy. Four cells, eight cells, they had doubled every day. Eight cells seemed huge, almost ready for the BabyBjörn. Then we would hang up, give each other fist bumps, curl together by the hearth of the TV.

Now, a nurse in a papery shower cap appeared. "Take off everything from the waist down and put this on." Usually they introduced themselves first, but today we got right down to brass tacks.

With a smile, No-Name Nurse handed me a square of thick, papery blanket. I took it without so much as a sigh. "Isn't Dr. Marion going to come give us the embryo report?"

"Yes, right before you're ready."

Despite our agreement that twins would be hard, Ken and I had barely discussed the prospect since the preop meeting. "No point counting our eggs before they hatch," he said.

"Ha. Good point," I said back.

The night before, we had finally weighed the odds: we would do IVF only once. Transferring two embryos upped our chances of getting one, instead of none, from 40 percent to 50 percent, which sounded solid, like a coin flip. It had come down to numbers, with Ken feverishly rambling about game-theory scenarios while I mused over what to wear to my impregnation.

Finally, he had come up with a suggestion, just as we'd convened in the cave. "How about if the odds of twins are less than 20 percent, we'll go ahead and put in two?"

"Fine," I'd agreed, reaching for the remote control, almost at the end of *Lost*. "Did we see this episode with the parallel world?"

They might be celebrating "infertility awareness" in the lobby of the clinic, but I was ready to bring mine to an end.

We waited for Dr. Marion.

"I guess I'm going to make a major life decision with my pants off," I said to Ken quietly. "On ten milligrams of Valium."

"I'm sure that's how a lot of people get knocked up," he said.

Then Dr. Marion whirled in. "Out of the seven awesome embryos, you've got one BB and one BC."

I had no idea what that meant, though I knew Ken had been trawling the Internet to understand these ratings. I figured all those Bs and Cs meant the same as they would in school—our two blasts were passing, while the other five had flunked.

She showed us black-and-white pictures. They already had an embryonic sac—which was as good as a soccer trophy for making them seem like kids.

"They're cute," I gushed.

"One hundred microns," Dr. Marion said.

"The width of a hair," Ken translated for me.

"I recommend putting them both in," Dr. Marion said. "It's a fifty percent chance of getting one, and a twenty percent chance of twins."

Those were the magic numbers—almost. Twenty percent represented the boundary but seemed close enough. We both laughed.

"What should we do?" I said to Ken.

"Okay?"

"Let's do it."

"Yeah."

Like that, we made the choice. The conversation took ten seconds, less time than I'd devoted to choosing Rice Krispies over raisin bran. We'd give our little B and C students a chance to be born.

I'd been diligent in filling my bladder, and the nurse now had me hobble to the bathroom to empty it. "Go for the count of four and then stop. Stand up if you have to." I held the gown closed, rushing past Suit Guy at the desk.

Back in the room, I had to put not my feet but my knees in the stirrups, so it wasn't as absurdly spread-eagle as it had first appeared. I took this as a positive sign, that I might negotiate the *degree* of discomfort and exposure, if not the frequency and necessity.

After some moments, the room filled—Ken, No-Name Nurse, Dr. Marion, and I were joined by two more women, who appeared together as a pair, mysteriously, from the back-room lab. The all-female makeup of the medical team seemed suddenly significant. It was like the Isle of Wonder Woman with fertility maenads.

I felt grateful to see smiles all around. We were not making love to conceive a baby. We were not two bodies in heat, twisting in unity toward an orgasm that would give new life. We were six people in a sterile room, and it meant a lot to me that the mood was upbeat—almost festive—if slightly strange. We were trying to make a baby, no matter how clinical, no matter the crowd. Forget it takes a village to raise a child. It takes a village to *make* a child.

As the procedure began, I floated above my body, less than half aware, an old habit I'd tried for years to unlearn. Now it came in handy, this ability to leave the ship when seas got rough.

Speculum, and then some kind of washing.

Dr. Marion's voice came next. "You'll feel this. It might feel cold. You'll feel something come out. It's supposed to. It's not the embryo coming out."

In went the thingy. Then the lab maenads brought out a needle and some fluid. For once I didn't dread the sight: our babies were swimming around in there—one sturdy blast, one a bit smaller.

I watched the black-and-white screen, which showed my uterus and the thin line of the catheter.

"Your uterus looks wonderful," Dr. Marion said. It felt like the finest compliment I'd ever received. "You have the perfect 'three layers.'" For implantation, the lining's thickness mattered.

I beamed.

In went the stuff, a little gush on the screen. For a

moment, no one spoke. A beat later, a second gush. Then more quiet.

"They landed perfectly," Dr. Marion told us.

I felt a rush of euphoria, like the best part of a favorite song played on high volume. I knew, for the first time and with absolutely no ambiguity, that I wanted these babies. Both, if I could. One, two, even three, should one of them split. In that moment the so-called burden of multiples didn't matter—I wanted the babies, our family. *I am pregnant now*, I realized. *I am finally pregnant.* It was a feeling of joy so intense it had physical power, like a shiver that kept going, and it lasted three whole days.

Week Four:

Fertility Feng Shui Squared

We didn't know which would come first—the sofa from Macy's or the phone call from Dr. Marion. I'd had the final blood draw one day before. After a restless night, I now tried to focus on the sofa, and on readying the downstairs room to which it would be delivered. The basement had always been tied up with babymaking. I had started clearing it out before the surgery to remove a fibroid, one that dangled from the top of my uterus like a chandelier.

The project had been a perfect distraction: time-sucking and physical. The floor was a cement slab that slanted toward a central drain. Unused pipe jutted from one wall. The room mirrored my womb with its unwelcome growth— due to irregular plumbing, people could not hang out there. For years the basement had harbored old junk, broken bookcases, stacked boxes. To take my mind off my terror of dying on a table beneath bright lights, I'd purged this room little by little, until it was empty. The week before the surgery, we'd put in clean, smooth hardwood floors.

For months it had stayed empty, until Ken got in on the feng shui attack. "We should put something there if it's going to be a rec room."

"How about a dark-colored sofa we could spill stuff on?"

To my surprise, he agreed.

Unbeknownst to Ken, I'd already been rearranging the house to invite a baby. I didn't want to offend his sensibilities as a scientist, a man who wrangled tiny photons through a large microscope. Like many physicists, though, he subscribed to the mystical, understood that in the quantum realm, the lines began to blur. He also harbored deep superstitions, once handed down in Yiddish, about what should and should not be spoken. Nevertheless, he'd accepted that my campaign to get a puppy included the premise that an animal would help lure a baby. Despite all this, he still believed the sperm needed to meet the egg for us to reproduce.

So, without explaining why, I'd cut down on the endless framed pictures of us as a couple. I thought a baby might not like the excessive celebration of our twosome, would feel like three was a crowd. Likewise, I clustered all our displays and knickknacks into "family" configurations, not pairs. I put two candlesticks with two salt and pepper shakers, two vases with two dishes. I carefully arrayed four trivets, since someday we'd find ourselves a family of four: Ken, Friso, a baby, and me. I figured everything in the environment should support this vision. In the backyard, I planted in fours: four snapdragons, four foxgloves. Lacking formal religion to structure my powerlessness, I defaulted to suburban animism.

In the last leg of IVF, the week of waiting for news, I managed to distract myself with Friso, who was finishing puppy obedience school. We'd do hours of "sit" and "down" commands, as if cramming for PhD orals. He would respond about half the time but seemed to prefer cuddling in our laps or sneaking off to the kitchen to poop in a corner.

I found that the Internet world had a name for this last stretch before the big verdict: "the two-week wait" or, in infertility chat rooms, "the tww." Its primary known side effect, agony, seemed to afflict almost everyone. For once I didn't bother searching my physical symptoms online. If those takeout dry-fried green beans made me queasy, it could be almost anything. I wouldn't allow a bunch of strangers online to get me riled.

Of course the new sofa and the call from Dr. Marion came at the same time. Two guys were downstairs, attaching wooden legs to an ottoman, when the phone rang. It seemed to happen in slow motion, the ring, the reach for the phone, the settling with Ken on our living room sofa. Our future was known—just not to us.

"I'm putting you on speaker," Ken said.

"Hi, guys," Dr. Marion said. I knew the news by her tone. "You are pregnant." She even drew out her words, speaking at an unexpectedly leisured pace. "Your HCG levels are off the charts," she continued, while we said back and forth, "Wow!" and, "Oh my God!" and, "We did it!"

When we hung up, we high-fived, hugged, and stared at each other with gawping fish mouths. Then we went downstairs and gave the sofa guys a fat tip. One of them handed us his card and asked us to write to his manager. By

noon we'd sent a glowing four-paragraph testimonial of
commendation, gushing about their delivery skills. Friso,
sensing the excitement, zoomed in loops through the room,
leaping on and off the sofa, attacking the new fabric with
paws and teeth.

"That little guy helped us get pregnant," I told Ken.
"Eighty percent puppy, twenty percent IVF."

"Dr. Marion would love that," he said.

And the salt and pepper shakers, I thought but did not say.

THREE DAYS LATER, we returned to the clinic for another
blood draw. It was too soon to see anything on an
ultrasound, but I still showed high amounts of HCG—
human chorionic gonadotropin, the pregnancy hormone—
nearly twice the "normal" amount.

No one said this might be an indicator of twins, though
of course it was. If I had a hunch, I squashed it. Through the
years of infertility, I'd worn myself out with "gut feelings"—
the exhausting and unreliable cousins of "hope." Now, I
assiduously did *not* think about the chest stabs of envy I'd
felt over Tina's twins, nor about the twin baby pictures
stashed around the house, Oprah-style "manifestation"
projects I'd long abandoned. It had been far less expensive
than the feng shui basement renovation to tear images from
magazines, and I'd lit on a set of glossy twins as "mine." I
glued them to a poster board—then took them off. I cut
them in half and pasted one baby back. *No way do I want
twins!* Yet I couldn't get rid of that cute second baby, so I
snuck him upstairs and stuck him into a remaining dis-

played photo of Ken and me, tucked into the frame's edge.

That was all irrelevant now, I reminded myself. We'd chosen hard science. From the doubled HCG, I simply granted myself a small serving of relief, that the number was unambiguous, that IVF had worked.

Dr. Marion had deemed carrying twins "high risk," but it seemed like something doctors loved to say, part of a vaguely punitive program aimed at making me feel nervous about something I couldn't control—for example, my age. The label felt as prohibitive as knowing that one in four people have serious car accidents. I still drove.

In that first week of confirmed conception, all I wanted was for the discomfort and drama to pass, the medical extravaganza to end. I didn't need a blood test to know my hormone levels were off the charts. The day after the call with the first HCG report, a single red bump had appeared on my clavicle, then spread upward onto my neck, morphing from the state of Florida downward onto my chest to become Texas. The blotch then resolved into individually clustered red dots, throbbing with itchiness and heat. They were angry dots, I thought—was I angry? What I felt was overloaded—with fear, longing, and exhaustion, all of it erupting onto my skin. Then the red blob appeared again, moving northward to colonize my jaw.

"We need to suppress the immune reaction," Dr. Marion said, meeting me in the clinic hallway, peering at my rash. "Otherwise your body could reject all foreign entities." Mere days into this pregnancy seemed too soon to have a complication. I stared forlornly at the carpet as she listed the drugs I should take. "Zantac, Benadryl, and prednisone."

"Isn't prednisone a steroid?" I pictured a boy born with meaty muscles, or a girl with a beard.

"It is, and it will reduce the swelling."

"Am I going to explode into puffiness?"

"Not at this dose," she reassured me. "You'll do 2.5 milligrams for three days, half that for two more."

"I don't want any more drugs," I whined, feeling a massive hangover from IVF, not to mention whatever the pregnancy was pumping through my veins. "Do I have to take this?"

Dr. Marion nodded. "My sister just called me with the same question. She'd been prescribed some things she didn't want to take, and she asked me if she had to take them. I told her she did. And you have to take this."

I surrendered. By sharing some snippet of her sibling life, my doctor saw me as a real person, I thought. I didn't feel like a real person, though, I felt like a collection of insane and insatiable impulses inhabiting a body no longer my own. The so-called "side effects" had become my central experience: fatigue, grumpiness, thirst. I guzzled bottle after bottle of smartwater, my throat like sandpaper.

Twelve hours of sleep passed like twelve minutes, and I felt like I was wearing sunglasses in a dim room while slurping Jack Daniel's from a bag. I thought with wonder of those people who didn't know they were pregnant for months. On television, women always snuck off to a bathroom to agonize over a home pregnancy kit, or they sprinted down the hall to throw up, then lifted their heads in dawning realization.

I had none of that, only the surprise of finding myself

suddenly reduced to physical sensations, all magnified like every episode of PMS I'd ever had, now unfolding in one grand, symphonic reprise. I no longer had the energy to rearrange the house or even watch TV. My thoughts dissolved only in sleep. When the persistent inkling arose that there might be more than one "foreign entity" aboard, I pressed it to the side of my roiling mind. Perhaps I even knew, though I did not trust myself.

It was in this state that Ken and I set off to Lake Tahoe for a family get-together, five days of seclusion with my father and stepmother. I did not consider how raw I truly felt, or that this visit might be hard. I couldn't wait to share our news.

WEEK FIVE:

A BABY WON'T FIX MY FAMILY, but TWINS MIGHT

At the resort in Lake Tahoe, Ken and I waited for my father and Belinda to arrive after a long flight from Florida. Meanwhile, we scoped out nearby restaurants, of which only a few were open in the May off-season. We picked a Polynesian place with a promising tofu dish—like Ken, I'd been a vegetarian for decades.

The venue, a five-minute walk from our door, looked perfect for a celebration. Though it was early in the pregnancy, and caution dictated we pause with our news at least until twelve weeks, I knew we'd tell them right away. Aside from the love-fest I expected after announcing the arrival of my father's first grandchild, I wanted to explain my bi-hourly megasnacks and why I practically chomped off my fingers getting through a Clif bar. I'd been passing out for the night at seven o'clock, a heavy-lidded narcoleptic plunge into mouth-breathing unconsciousness. Then there were the long naps and the neck rash, the pills and the water. We'd known about the pregnancy for only four days, but already it wasn't shaping up to be subtle.

Hours later, we rallied my father and stepmother to the restaurant's outdoor entrance. I felt anxious to sit down and dazzle them with our reproductive success, and hungry enough to rip the menu from the glass door and gnaw it. In the chilly dusk, my father and Belinda stared at the posted specials in silence.

"It looks a little expensive," my father said.

"This is a resort, in a tourist town," I pointed out.

"Fusion? 'Fusion' is French for 'overpriced.'"

"There's not much nearby, and we're pretty hungry." The last thing I wanted to do was drive around Tahoe to find a Chevys. Despite the Friso-like whimper welling within me, I thought our condition merited the convenience—or would once they knew.

After more quiet, my father turned to Belinda. "We'll split something?"

She shrugged. They followed us inside.

I guzzled a glass of water right away and asked for another, while my father and Belinda continued to study the menu with glazed eyes. We hadn't even been together for an hour, and already I'd let them down, missed some cue from the culture of their tightly bound twosome. They always picked up the dinner tab, and I didn't understand their tension.

Their straight lips bent to frowns. My father was not living precariously, though he did like to joke that his favorite brand was "En Salé." A retired lawyer, he and my stepmother, once his secretary, traveled the world together, popping to Paris, cruising around Italy. She was blonde, Southern, outspoken: a woman who usually got her way. I'd been close to Belinda in childhood, through which she'd showered me with affection and polo shirts. Somehow we'd drifted apart, each of us into the separate satellites of our so-called blended family.

She had four children from three marriages, and four grandchildren. The entire gang of them visited my father and Belinda regularly in Naples, Florida, or all of them tromped off to North Carolina for a weeklong party of crab-hammering dinners, boisterous banter, inside jokes, and beach portraits where everyone went barefoot and wore white. My sister and I hadn't been invited to the most recent bash.

"We assumed you wouldn't come," my father had said.

"It wouldn't have hurt to ask," I'd replied, knowing he was right and hating how I felt like an artifact, a vestige. Sometimes, just the word "family" made my voice crack. I knew it should evoke the notion of togetherness, but sometimes it felt more like separate, stressful camps.

Now, here I was in Tahoe, with a fresh and fragile pregnancy, hormones seeping from my sweaty skin. I was thirty-nine, happily married, yet it took me only a moment of their hemming and hawing about the price of food to bring up ancient feelings about my parents' long-ago divorce, about being left behind. What might have passed with a wince was now magnified by the hunger-thirst-sleepiness and an expectation that was both pervasive and unnamed: that somehow being pregnant would heal the relationships in my own family of origin. Even without their knowing, this child within me would caulk the cracks. Belinda would adore me again, and my father would be further bound to me by forces of biology. I wanted a cathartic reunion. Meanwhile, they probably just wanted a burger. So much of family relationships comes down to this: one person is pining for recognition, while the other, oblivious, simply craves a sandwich.

"I guess we'll have that tofu dish, too," my father said. They were not vegetarians and generally mocked soy. "We'll split it. And we'll split one glass of chardonnay."

We gave the waiter our orders with a maximum lack of enthusiasm, as if selecting loaves from a Soviet bread line. Then, finally, I nodded to Ken. He would deliver the actual words.

"We have some exciting news." He paused for drama. "We. Are. Expecting."

I bit my lip shyly, brimming with pride. I hadn't yet managed to say it in the first-person singular: *I am expecting.* It seemed more manageable to think we'd share the task, the way my parents were sharing dinner. If it were I alone, perhaps I'd lose the baby, but not if Ken were pregnant, too. Not that we said "pregnant," either—it seemed so presumptuous, so dauntingly physical.

"Oh my goodness," my father said, finally smiling. He lifted their wine. They brought energy into their jet-lagged voices, proclaiming joy despite glassy-eyed expressions.

"It's still early in the pregnancy, isn't it?" Belinda asked.

"It is," Ken said.

"I can't tell yet what's pregnancy and what's recovering from IVF. You can probably see this rash." I stroked my red, blotchy neck.

"Amy did that so many times," she said, meaning IVF. "It was horrendous." Amy was Belinda's only daughter, my stepsister, who had ended up adopting. My stepmother sounded wistful, distant, as if somehow my pregnancy only brought her back to her own child's pain. Or perhaps this was meant as a bid for common ground, but instead I felt my presence recede, my body given over to primordial tasks, my mind dimmed down with nagging fear.

I, too, had new perspective on Amy's struggle, but I didn't see what it had to do with me, or I didn't want to. Though recently I'd been a grudging avoider of all things baby, I had already forgotten how much someone else's pregnancy could bring feelings of less than bliss.

THAT FIRST NIGHT IN THE SIERRAS, I drank three tall bottles of smartwater and still felt parched. I'd been warned in dire terms to stay slaked; one clinic nurse had named dehydration as the leading cause of miscarriage. My throat was a desiccated plant that would never be revived from its crusty wilt. Plastic containers piled up by the bed. I gasped all night, clutching each bottle of water, and woke up to a snowy view from our window—a central pool area draped in white.

We were all stuck inside.

"Do you want to walk to the casino?" my father asked.

"I can't be around smoke," I said.

"We could walk around the lake," Belinda suggested.

"It's snowing out," I croaked. "I can barely get out of bed."

They stared at me, and I tried to grasp again that my pregnancy didn't mean my family would suddenly devote themselves to the doting for which I longed. Belinda went off by herself to the spa, and my father left to find her a Mother's Day gift. We'd brought her a bottle of Sonoma cabernet, but it turned out she drank only white. My father got her a pot of yellow dahlias, and, as if we were in parallel worlds, Ken took me to a nearby shop and bought me a fuzzy fleece. Later, my father went with Belinda to the casino, where they lost $80.

In the evening, I ended up alone with Belinda in the shared living room—Ken and my dad were off fetching personal pizzas for a stay-at-home dinner. I decided I needed to explain how hard it had been, that for years we hadn't conceived, and that IVF had left me feeling ill.

"Amy got pregnant a few times with IVF but miscarried," Belinda said. My stepmother, who had her own first kid at eighteen, clearly didn't put much stock in our petridish prospects.

"Hmm," I said, not wanting to discuss the m-word.

"It was terrible."

"I'm sure."

In this way, my infertility and IVF experiences prepared me for carrying twins: people's comments would come uncensored. Likewise, I would never be sure if my sense of offense expanded in the heat of hormones, or whether insensitivity was simply commonplace. The two possibilities could not be separated any more than I could walk out into the Tahoe blizzard and parse hydrogen and oxygen from the snow blast in my face.

Or maybe my aggravation in that moment was another post-divorce syndrome, sibling competition, I versus the stepsister who got my dad. My original one-baby plan had evolved in part from the idea that my child would have the world to him or herself. Either way, I had a yearning to celebrate my hard-won pregnancy. I hoped that this second Amy comparison was the end of it, but the next afternoon, it came up again.

"Did you get any extra embryos?" Belinda asked.

"We had two good ones, and they put them both in."

"Any extras?"

"No."

"That's too bad—then you'd have another chance if this pregnancy doesn't work out."

Of course she was right. Her personal experience, not to mention statistical reality, bolstered her concern. I had opened the topic of IVF. Still, I raised my hand in the stop position. "I don't even want to talk about this. We feel lucky we got what we did." Later, Belinda would claim I "wagged a finger in her face," but I was only trying to shield myself, not lecture.

After that, there was more than thirst keeping me up that night. I desperately wanted my parents to *get it*, the force and frailty of our possible dream. Instead, we were perusing the potential grief of miscarriage. Wasn't this supposed to be a vacation? The very idea of "vacation" seemed preposterous in my terrified state. I'd been pregnant only a bunch of days, but already it wasn't what I'd thought. First the rash, now this. Where was the joy? Only when I closed the door, to find myself alone with Ken, did I remember we were lucky, we'd gotten where we'd tried to go. I watched videos of Friso at his day care posted on Facebook, and I cried as I thought,

My baby, my baby. On top of the stress I already felt, I worried that the stress itself would cause exactly what everyone kept mentioning—miscarriage. The next morning, I obsessed about getting home, but the snow fell in thick, stagey billows, coating the streets white. I made continuous calls about getting snow tires, talked to the front desk about the road closings.

"But when do you *think* they might open?" I asked, as if they secretly knew how to stop the snow.

"Not for at least another day," they said.

I slept for eighteen hours.

At the next breakfast, I croaked over my tea. If only I could make them understand how I felt, they would rush in to nurture me. "I don't know if it's the IVF or the pregnancy or the drugs I'm taking now, but I still feel like shite."

Belinda looked up from the stove, where she'd been making bacon for herself and my father. "Amy went through this. It was a total emotional roller coaster. It worked at first, and then, all of sudden, gone."

Something snapped. I couldn't hear one more time about someone else's terrible loss. "I don't want to talk about Amy. My situation is different. I feel like you guys are waiting for me to have a miscarriage."

"Kathy!" my father barked.

"Well, it's true."

"It's not true, and it's offensive."

"You keep bringing it up."

Belinda stormed out.

I returned to our room, looked out the window at the blizzard of white. Later, my father would claim I'd said they were "hoping" for a miscarriage—which I knew I never would have said, nor did I believe.

For the rest of the trip, Belinda sat listlessly before a television in the main room, watching *The Blind Side*, while, a few feet away, my dad and Ken played cards. I joined them at the table, slurping tea. None of us spoke much, and the movie filled the space, the story of a lost boy finally finding family.

We left right after the snow melted, a day earlier than planned. The feeling in the condo hadn't thawed a bit. My father and Belinda walked us out to our car.

"Thanks for taking care of us," I said to Belinda, hoping we could bluff ourselves to a moment's truce.

"It seems like you take care of yourself," she said flatly, the two of us frozen in a stiff half hug, as if fused in mutual misunderstanding.

Finally, stepping into the shotgun seat, I was able to exhale. I'd never been happier to be headed home. There, I stewed for a day, then tried to smooth things over by phone. My father and I argued over what had been said. He didn't believe that Belinda had asked about extra embryos, and I remembered that was how it goes in a family, that facts can fade faster than feelings.

"We were nothing but excited for you. We even talked about it. What if you have *twins*?" He seemed moved by the prospect. Maybe that's what it would take: not one baby, but two.

WEEK SIX:

WE ARE THRILLED! RiGHT?

In the waiting room of the clinic, no one looked directly at anyone, though glances darted sidelong from behind old *Esquires* and *Vogues*. I, too, felt unable to resist peeking at the other women, and I pondered the infertility treatment uniform everyone had come to independently: loose tops, flip-flops, sweats. A stretchy waistband was easy on a bruised belly, and flip-flops came off fast. I looked down at my own exposed toes, painted pink. When you see your feet in stirrups almost daily, the dash of color can be cheering.

At 9:10, I whispered to Ken, "I can't stand it."

He squeezed my hand.

"The waiting," I said, squirming. "Why are they so late?"

"Ten minutes," Ken said.

"If they don't call us back in five, let's leave and find another doctor."

"Okay," Ken said. "That's a good idea."

At 9:12, a nurse with a clipboard called my name.

I walked stiffly, trying not to vibrate with our recent

good news. I still identified with the other women there, still despised those who over the years had gloated at their random feats of reproductive luck. Besides, my excitement hummed with fear, a loud voice in the choir that couldn't hold the happy tune. Now that I was "pregnant"—if I was indeed still "pregnant"—how did I know the baby would stick? It was a tiny camper bivouacked on the side of my uterus, perched precariously in the dark. Maybe its little tent had come unstaked. Maybe this was like the delusional pregnancies of the past three years, episodes of PMS spent trawling the Internet to study lists of "early symptoms," or squinting at one-lined pee sticks by a window.

At last, the nurse escorted us to a back room. "Undress from the waist down," she said, the phrase they always used —a request but also a command, reminding you the next stage of waiting would involve being half-naked. "The doctor will be in soon."

Though I knew the drill, the transition from pregnant person to pantsless patient spiked my adrenaline. I wore my favorite jeans and a red down vest—both already snug. I'd been avoiding the sweatpants uniform, and denim was like my skin, only tougher. In my armor of blue canvas, I felt in charge—"wearing the pants." I'd been wearing the same pair since Tahoe, and shed them now with great reluctance.

I hadn't gotten used to this disrobing, placing my bare butt on the paper mat. If anything, it got cumulatively more humiliating. I'd once assumed that if you suffer something enough, over time it gets easier. I now recognized this idea as another flavor of denial, especially in regard to others, and to women in particular. *It's her second round of cancer. She must know the chemo routine. That's the way it is for her.* Instead, some difficult things stayed difficult.

The paper on the exam chair reminded me of the waxy sheets used to wrap sandwiches at the deli. Here, at this private clinic run mostly by women, they at least offered actual sheets to cover up, so you didn't have to cower like Eve with nothing but a cocktail napkin. Like the pink toenails, I grasped at small bits of solace.

"Why can't they make an IVF cruise?" I asked Ken. "We'd sleep on a big boat. Shots would happen by the pool, with blood draws by the casino."

"We'd try our odds in every sense."

"Exactly. Anyone who gets pregnant could vomit over the side rail."

"Then go straight to the buffet to reload."

Our banter distracted me from my antsiness for only a moment. It was the opposite of sex: once you take your pants off, the action stops. Every minute felt like twenty. I studied the decor: the ballerina mobile dangling overhead, the striped socks on the stirrups, the dimming lampshade, the plaid curtain. I appreciated that they kept the rubber gloves tidy, so they didn't look like disembodied hands, and the lube wasn't lying around, like there'd been a big orgy. I clutched at these visuals, as if less exposed when judging the furnishings. Whatever happened that day, I told myself, I could soon get back to natural remedies: yoga, juice, magical thinking. I could finally get off the medical mill.

"I can't stand it," I said. If the news was bad, I wanted it *now*—a kosher killing of hope, one quick slash. "Let's leave."

"Okay." Ken squeezed my hand again. He'd come to

every appointment, fielded every phone call. He'd run to Pharmaca for Valium, for ice packs, for Coconut Bliss. He'd walked Friso and ordered the Chinese, gassed up my car and rubbed my feet. But only I could be the one to take yet another test.

"Any minute now," he said.

"Maybe you should take your pants off, too, in solidarity."

"Ha ha."

Dr. Marion whirled in, breathless. "Let's switch rooms. The machine next door is better."

She handed me a sheet to drape around my bare behind, and we hustled one room over. Ken carried my jeans, purse, and puffy vest.

I left my body for the wanding procedure, never used to the invasion of equipment, and focused on the black-and-white fuzzy screen. All three of us were riveted—it could have been a landing on Mars.

As I sprawled on my back again, Ken held my hand and also jammed three fingers against my ribs, a pressure that helped distract from the discomfort of the ultrasound—another tiny trick.

Lines and dots appeared, and I thought, *Okay, it's still there.* I turned back to the ceiling, exhaled.

Dr. Marion and Ken were silent, the kind of silence that filled a room with noise, like static.

"Is that what I think it is?" Ken asked, with an optical physicist's skill for reading grainy images.

"Yes, it is," Dr. Marion answered.

"What?" I asked, trying to maintain my status as half in my body but following the screen.

"You have twins," Dr. Marion said, in a neutral tone, with none of the excitement from the "you're pregnant" call.

"Oh my God." My eyes locked on Ken's. His hands had come off my ribs.

We were thrilled!

Right?

"They are about the size of a grain of rice."

When the ultrasound was over, no one spoke.

Ken broke the silence. "Wow."

My head bobbled, as if this information physically weighted my brain.

Dr. Marion did not shout down the hall for non-alcoholic champagne. She folded her arms, waiting for us, while we waited for her. Even after this news, we were still waiting, this time for words. Then, when we said nothing, she launched into details of my twin pregnancy regimen.

"You need to eat six hundred extra calories a day. Don't read *What to Expect When You're Expecting*—read only the section on vegetarianism. As for exercise, you want to do about sixty percent of your regular routine."

I nodded, as if these numbers were all I needed to know.

She reeled off more facts, and all I could think was, *Twins*. The sound of it felt empty, rather than double. Dr. Marion and Ken kept looking at me *as if this were actually happening*. We'd signed something about this. I'd gushed about love and miracles. But shouldn't a miracle feel more . . . exciting? What was wrong with me? God was raining manna, times *two*, and I was fretting over excess carbs.

From that moment forward, people would be asking if we were surprised to have twins, and the answer would be a genuine "yes." Despite our having done IVF and transferred two embryos, it came as a shock. It was kind of like opening a credit card bill and finding out your spending added up to *that*. It's all the more stunning to recognize you did it all yourself.

Mostly, though, it didn't feel real. It would have been the same if a clown in full whiteface had sprinted down the hall of the fertility clinic—I would have thought, *Weird, surprising, scary*—possibly *fun*, but mostly *baffling*.

Dr. Marion kept talking. "I also need to tell you there's something called vanishing-twin syndrome. About twenty percent of the time, one just vanishes."

"The syndrome is well named," Ken said, to say something.

I nodded, fairly sure this would happen to us. Wasn't 20 percent our number now? I didn't feel happy or sad. It was simple math. One would disappear, like those second lines on the pregnancy test stick through the years of infertility. First there were two, but when you looked again, it was really only one.

"You have a ninety-three percent chance of a live birth of one baby." Through the haze of my numbness, Dr. Marion struck me as almost apologetic.

"It's amazing," I said, not sure if I wanted to reassure her, or Ken, or myself.

We got the printout of the ultrasound, which I could interpret much more clearly now with my butt covered. I gaped at the evidence. In a sea of scratchy black, thin white lines circumscribed two dots—the heart of each baby.

Dr. Marion studied my jeans. "You won't be wearing those much longer."

I knew it was true, but for once, I wasn't worrying about my pants, riveted instead by the glossy photo in my hand, by the double omelet in black and white.

I headed with Ken to the parking lot, where we collided, arms wrapped, thick throated, and kissed—not exactly a passionate kiss, but one urgent with all that hadn't yet been spoken, or perhaps even felt.

I kept thinking of the strain in Dr. Marion's face, which seemed more significant than what she'd said.

"Stay off the Internet," she had warned, sending us off with hugs. Did she know something about this whole twin thing that I didn't? At least for a while, it was better not to know.

WEEK SEVEN:

Vaginal Lady Central

For the next week, Ken and I didn't talk much about this major development—that by the end of IVF, I was pregnant with twins. In the passing moments it felt real, it seemed perilous and uncertain. By then I knew that my stepmother, who'd so upset me asking about the pregnancy's permanence, had merely voiced my own fears. There was no reason to assume things would go well, especially now, with multiples. I couldn't discuss it with Ken. I did not trust myself with the news. If I voiced any angst about having two, then something bad might happen to one or both. If I reveled in twins, that, too, could magnetize misfortune. The pregnancy felt like a tenaciously lurking stray cat, back again for milk, this time with a furry friend. We couldn't quite call them ours. We'd just feed them both and see.

Ken's superstition also dictated a degree of nondiscussion, or maybe we both needed a pause in the stress. Either way, we simply put the black-and-white ultrasound in our dining room, propped against a wedding photo that had survived the fertility feng shui purge. I stared at them every day, two sacs, two hearts. I slept from early evening to late morning, walked Friso as far as I could, sometimes over an hour. I distributed flyers for our neighborhood earthquake association, huffing and puffing after climbing one or two stairs, Friso pulling me along.

I followed Dr. Marion's order not to trawl the Internet. Online infertility forums were shark-infested waters of dashed hopes and worst cases. In cyberspace, people who represented the negative-outcome percentages gathered to grieve in intimate anonymity. Women signed their names above lists of treatments and dates of miscarriages, as if these were advanced degrees on a résumé. I certainly understood the impulse, but reading those posts could leave me paralyzed for days. The electronic chatter about twin pregnancy might be just as grim.

Instead of reading about possible problems of double gestation, I decided to get out of the house. I would breathe fresh air, bask in the great yellow ball of Prozac in the sky. One day, after walking Friso to panting exhaustion, I decided I would do something else, something symbolic and positive: face down the Vagina Ladies at a nearby baby boutique.

A Vagina Lady is anyone who overshares the details of her childbirth experience and its aftermath. Soon after I married Ken, at a Christmas party in San Francisco, I met my first. The men had gathered by the cheese dip to talk about sci-fi movies, while a group of women clustered by the dessert table. As we loaded our napkins with sweets, one of our group started in on dilation and epidurals, a zealous monologue that commanded complete quiet from the rest of us. I stood there in my black tights and black boots, nibbling a Santa-shaped cookie, while she reminisced about her cervix and asked, "Any of you have an episiotomy?"

"Ugh, yes," said one of the others. I tuned out. As the only childless woman in that circle, I had nothing to contribute about the state of my vagina and the road conditions after heavy traffic. Even then, when I still assumed things would be easy, I didn't like the idea of being defined by birth and its gore. Or perhaps I sensed what was to come. Either way, during the years of infertility, these Vagina Ladies, as Ken and I called them, became even harder to bear.

There was a kids' store in Berkeley's Gourmet Ghetto neighborhood where they seemed to cluster, a store with everything organic, BPA-free, or made of wood. I often made last-minute pit stops there for gifts. Airy and small, the boutique always had at least two women in rapt conversation, drooling babies in their arms. One woman was always breastfeeding, and the other had a toddler. They each had long hair in a low ponytail and generally evinced little interest in the shopper, though I deduced at least one of them worked there. I thought they could sense I didn't have a child and stared right through me. This was another side effect of infertility: when so much *doesn't* happen, you start to imagine other kinds of stuff.

"That place smells like diapers and stale breast milk," I would complain to Ken, though it was my own discomfort that wafted on the air. "It's Vagina Lady central." More and more, I had rushed past it as if those displays of monkey bibs and stuffed giraffes were bricks of uranium.

Now, one week after learning I was pregnant with twins,

I decided to enter this humming hive of mommies. I intended to buy a gift for a pregnant neighbor, another person I'd avoided. For years she and her husband had been congregating with their first child in front of our house. Getting my period would almost force them to materialize. The approach of their chubby-cheeked daughter came with the *Jaws* soundtrack.

Now, we were pregnant together, and I figured I could enter a baby store without a pinched throat and dizzied vision. I could paw the receiving blankets and miniature pants without a feeling of panic and alienation. It would help solidify this thing the doctors were telling me: pregnant, with twins. Not *one* baby, but *two*. Inside me. Growing. Screaming for pancakes.

In the store, a brunette approached, her baby in a sling. "Can I help?"

I stood at a table of pint-size tops, suddenly blanking on my gift-buying mission, overwhelmed by the prospect that these clothes could be filled with *babies*. Not any babies, but the ones Ken and I had made.

I nodded, and that dislodged a bulge in my throat. It floated up my neck, like a ball of wax rising in a lava lamp. "I just found out I'm pregnant," I croaked.

"Congratulations!"

"With twins. Twins." Suddenly the tears uncorked, along with a sob. "I don't know what to do with two."

"Do you have other kids?" she asked, unfazed by this sudden shift from my possibly buying a tiny $30 shirt to the revelation of my most personal fears.

"No," I whispered.

"That's good. I totally understand. I recently had my third, and it wasn't planned." She bounced up and down with her little packet.

I could hardly say ours were unplanned. My husband had contributed his DNA to a plastic cup in a bathroom filled with magazines and videos while I submitted to general anesthesia for surgery on my ovaries. We'd been cheering these creations along since they were four cells old. Still, I offered my most sincere response: "It's a shock."

"It's really big news."

"I'm really happy about it," I said. My eyes leaked more tears. "It's just . . ."

"I know, I know, I know. Here, sit here for as long as you need to." This woman with her sleepy newborn hanging from her front, this women who had seemed like a Vagina Lady ringleader—which in Berkeley is a serious title—led me to a glider in the corner of the room. "This is very soothing."

And it was. The funky gray maternity chair with dirty white piping had the most wonderful forward-and-back motion. I sat there rocking. A bunch of other people came and went while I rested. When I finally got up, I felt calmer. "I'm also here to buy a gift for a friend."

The shopkeeper nodded, again gracefully switching back from life crisis to consumer guide. I bought some footy pajamas with green frogs, and a soft red hat. I also picked out two infant hats for us—one with elephants in blue, yellow, and brown, and one with dinosaurs in red and blue.

"Are you having boys?" she asked.

"I don't know. These would work for either, don't you think?"

"Definitely," she agreed kindly, and then wrapped the present as I tucked the hats into my purse. At home, I kept them out in view, setting them on my grandmother's rocking chair in the nursery. The nursery. We were saying that now, rather than using the "second bedroom" label we had carefully cultivated.

I stared at those two hats. I couldn't help realizing how strange it was that these women who had seemed like "the enemy" during my infertility were suddenly the kind strangers who would *get it* even more than many of my friends, because after friends had listened to me complain for years, they would of course assume twins were nothing but an embarrassment of riches. Which they were.

SO AFTER I HAD TOLD a random woman in a kids' store, I told a woman pushing a double stroller on Solano Avenue, the shopping drag a few blocks from home. She was kind enough to stop and congratulate me, telling me the experience would be amazing. "The first year is hard, but I wouldn't trade it for anything. My advice is, get as much help as you can afford. You can't do it without help. But it is wonderful." Her daughters, as if on cue, looked cherubic in their seats, blue eyes twinkling over applesauce smiles.

Having told two complete strangers, around town, if not on the Internet, I figured it was time to tell my mother. So far I'd been greeted with compassion and enthusiasm. My mother could not be anything but thrilled. Right? Just like I was thrilled!

Over the phone, Berkeley to Bethesda, I delivered the news to silence.

"Wooowwww," she said.

"Yep," I said, acknowledging the shock of it and wishing for something more from her—excitement, perhaps, so that I could borrow some for myself.

She said nothing else, so I filled the gap. "Of course, it's still early. Sometimes one twin . . . vanishes. It's calling vanishing-twin syndrome." Why did I say this? I sounded apologetic, as if I'd done something rash, bought two cars.

"I'm going to tell Jenna," she said. Her assistant was there that day, filing papers. "Wow," she said when she came back. "Did . . . you . . . take any drugs?"

A few years earlier, I'd told her we were trying to conceive, but nothing more of our struggle. "We had a little help," I said, hoping she'd leave it at that. I didn't want to revive the topic of backup IVF embryos—no spare grandkids waiting on ice.

She didn't push. "You're going to need a lot of stuff. You should try to get things secondhand."

"Yeah," I said.

I was only beginning to ponder the financial implications of double baby. Having two at once meant we wouldn't have the benefit of hand-me-downs. Every expense, from pre-school to college, would hit us twice.

"What about Larry and Karen?" she asked, naming Ken's brother and his wife. "Maybe you can get cribs from them."

"Their girls are teenagers now. I doubt they still have cribs."

"Huh. Who else in Ken's family has kids?"

"Since Ken and I are so late to the party, most of the

goodies have been redistributed. Our friends are on their second child."

"There's always consignment."

"Or we can cruise around garbage night until we find a crib."

She didn't hear my sarcasm. "Lots of ways to find a bargain."

Twin pregnancy wasn't hurling me into a state of responsibility but was instead causing me to regress to a childish mode of materialism. I needed *stuff* to fill the gaps— lots of it, it seemed, as if parenting two infants would come down to the props. I had hoped such things would magically appear. My mother had the opposite idea—that this fact of twins more than anything meant I now needed to get in gear. That it was time to fight, time to scramble. But all I wanted to do was nap.

I hadn't yet told enough people about the twin factor to realize that I was entering a subculture, the way my mother had been in a minority as a single parent at the start of the divorce craze. Things would be harder than on the standard path. Twins were, in the words of another twin-mom acquaintance, "two for the price of three." That price was more than money.

On the phone with my mother, I felt strangely bereft and thoroughly unmaternal. Her nervous ambivalence mirrored mine precisely. Then my tiredness kicked into high gear and I felt kind of achy, wanting so much more from this talk, without even knowing what. My face felt hot, my hands strangely sore.

"I'm going to go now," I said.

"Okay—bye, sweetie."

What had I done? I curled back on the sofa. I had two new people inside me, and I'd never felt more alone.

My mother was telling me something other women would not: I would have to be resourceful. My entire world would shift, even before the babies came. Some friends, even close ones, long-term ones, would vanish into a mist. Others, in some cases people I hardly knew, would step forward to tirelessly offer their love and support. I didn't yet know who would fall into which camp, but I was beginning to see why it might be easier just to share things online.

Week Eight:

The Abrams Plan, and Hamburgers in Bed

We graduated from the fertility clinic with one last printed ultrasound, our double-major diploma in black and white. On the way out, already an insufferable parent, I showed the front-desk woman our two tiny blobs while careful to keep my voice to a low whisper, in deference to women waiting nearby. "Look at this!"

"Keep us posted," she said, with bored good cheer, our miracle now another receipt to file. Then she handed us our final bill. The postpregnancy scans, unlike the rest of IVF, weren't prepaid.

We would launch prenatal care, our first step toward the Promised Land of Pregnancy, though we'd be immigrants there, infertility refugees: uncertain of our status, wary of the customs, and doubting we could stay. Our insurance at least acknowledged pregnancy as a condition, unlike infertility. They would have covered a sex-change operation, according to the fine print, but not IVF—they'd pay for a penis, but not a baby. Now we had two on the way (babies, that is). Financial relief of insurance aside, I feared the excess exams that twins would require, knowing full well my "advanced age" made me "high risk," and "high risk" meant *please take off your pants and wait.*

Somewhere in my twenties, I stopped going to the gynecologist. I didn't believe that pap smears helped anything, except the likelihood I'd get the "abnormal" call, only to find after weeks of contemplating where my cremains should be scattered that everything was fine. It wasn't like going to the (also dreaded) dentist, where they at least maintained my mouth. An OB just snooped. To me, my private parts were "private," and also an ecosystem—say, a rain forest—that might have seasonal changes but in the end would cycle back to itself.

Every other year, I'd conduct a blitz of pants-on interviews with various reputable Bay Area gynecologists. Sometimes we'd chat in an actual exam room, but the fluorescent lights and the angle of those stirrups set off small, silent sirens in the depths of my brain, and even as I shook hands with whomever I'd interviewed, I'd think, *No fucking way, and goodbye forever.* I knew my fears were irrational, my inaction unwise, but that kind of logic and avoidance simply built on itself.

I had explained myself to Ken. "All they're going to do is give me tests, which will lead to more tests. Then, after the very the last one, they'll be like, 'Your uterus is a trapezoid.' Then they'll want to cut me open, and I'll be in the medical chute forever."

"That sounds kind of extreme," he'd say mildly, never one to pressure.

It was. In addition to being paranoid and immature, it turned out to be strangely prescient.

FOR THE YEARS BEFORE IVF, I'd seen a celebrated acupuncturist, whom I'll call Liza. It had taken months to get my first appointment, and there were typically three-hour waits for a fifteen-minute slot. We were mostly women, up to a dozen, gathered in the foyer of Liza's Marin mansion, nibbling oatmeal cookies and sipping chamomile tea. We settled awkwardly on her teak furniture, among fine orchids and Buddhist statuary, all of us huddled with laptops and phones, a quiet crowd of tapping supplicants.

Finally, as an afternoon or morning drifted by, Liza would appear in flowing black clothes, traipsing barefoot over her Persian carpets. With her mug of goopy green beverage in hand, she would pluck us one by one from purgatory. Sometimes, just getting to the treatment room felt cathartic. I allowed her to needle the soles of my feet and the pink of my gums, and smiled patiently if she took a cell phone call in the middle of our session.

"Sorry," she said once, when she came back. "My husband and I are closing on a house in France."

None of this discouraged me, neither the waiting nor the interruptions nor the massive expense—I believed the cumulative tension of those things would yield equivalent results. A "natural" approach had to be better, and I was high on hope, inhaling every wisp. "The doctor looks for the problem, whereas an acupuncturist creates a solution," I said to Ken on nights after Liza's, vigorous in my propaganda.

He shrugged. "If it helps you, then okay."

"You help me," I said, grateful again that he didn't push those maniacs, the Western doctors with their pills, shots, wands, and scalpels.

It took over a year for me to finally break down and start the standard fertility tests. Those ultimately revealed a fibroid that had doubled the size of my uterus, making it, in fact, shaped like a trapezoid. It also blocked both fallopian tubes, like homegrown birth control. It had to come out.

After that, the *right* doctor became my grail, Yelp the portal to an online underworld of extreme opinion. I wanted someone, preferably a woman, who could be as sensitive as a good friend, as wise as a beloved aunt. My hypothetical dream MD would like me a bit more than her other patients, but not in a weird way. I wanted my OB also to exude success, like Liza, because a healer should be someone who had clout with the universe. Fortune begets fortune, and some would rub off on me, on us, as we entered her orbit. I wanted my medical doctor to be part shaman, with the ability to prescribe Valium.

Of course, all these requirements safely kept me from actually visiting an OB, like a woman who wouldn't settle down unless she could marry George Clooney. Yet somehow, by the time it became clear I needed surgery on my misshapen womb, I finally found Dr. Abrams. My time with Liza paid off. "He's one of the only good ones," she said, giving me his name. "You'll be in good hands."

Ken came with me to the meet and greet, both of us shaking hands with a healthy-looking, California-fied, fifty-ish man with a charmingly curved nose, blondish, thinning hair and bright blue eyes. He wasn't a stare-at-his-clipboard guy but instead looked at our faces, as if he could see us as people, not as a pile of symptoms with a PPO, or one more couple who had waited too long. Despite the clinical setting, he had acted as if our interview were a small party in his home and we were the guests with whom he'd most prefer to linger.

"You will definitely have a baby. The only question is when and how," he said, no hedging, not even with the word "hopefully." I'd found my woman, and I didn't care if she was a man.

NOW, WHEN I WAS eight weeks along with two babies on board, Dr. Abrams blustered into the waiting room of his San Francisco OB practice. "Congratulations!" He gave both Ken and me huge hugs. "Twins—what a blessing."

Relief softened my body, and the waiting room blurred to soft focus. I longed for those words—for affirmation, for reassurance, to temper my own uncertainty.

Since this meeting would be a pure strategy session, he led us to a side room without a pit stop at the scale or the blood pressure cuff. I had no idea how much I weighed. I still wore my jeans, though with the top button undone. Once seated, I tucked into my Egg Mit sandwich from Noah's, the sensation of butter and bread in my mouth temporarily distracting me from the general malaise of hormones and fatigue. My skin had cleared up since Tahoe, except for one welt on my clavicle, a radioactive roach, like a lingering grudge.

I continued to wake at midnight to chomp on apples, cheese, and trail mix and dragged every day, even after thirteen hours of sleep. Once or twice, I'd found myself sobbing into Friso's back on the bathroom floor, asking Ken, "How will we care for this puppy with two babies?" as if this were the biggest challenge we faced.

"I'm going to give you the basic Abrams plan," our doctor said. He marked a piece of blank computer paper with small, neat print. Near the top, he wrote, "100 grams of protein a day," which, for a vegetarian and former caffeinetarian, was no small task. For a moment, I reeled back from my bagel. "You are to include protein at every meal. When you have a snack, like a piece of toast, load it with peanut butter."

"What about an apple?" I said, not at my smartest.

"Yes."

"A banana?"

"Peanut butter for that, too." He continued to narrate our plan of attack, how at week thirty-eight, we'd storm the compound and seize those babies. By C-section, that was— my fibroid surgery meant no natural birth. It seemed impossibly far in the future, and after a pulse of worry about the logistics of getting two babies out through my abdomen, I kicked that can down the road.

The plan went way beyond Dr. Marion's reading list. Monthly, then biweekly, and finally weekly, I would visit this office. Further, I would have at least monthly appointments with a perinatologist—whatever that was—which would similarly accelerate to possibly daily "non-stress tests," which sounded quite stressful. Those would monitor fetal heartbeats.

"Every *week* at the end?" I licked the poppy seeds off my knuckles. Like the butter marks darkening my jeans, the realization was sinking in: this was even more pants-off time on doctors' tables than I'd imagined. Despite shunning the Internet, I knew from peeking into books about multiples that a host of things could go wrong. I had accepted that I wasn't going to be giving birth at home in a plastic tub in the yard while Ken grilled soy burgers for the midwife. Still, I'd thought at least some part of the pregnancy would seem . . . natural.

I'd gone to see Liza right after Tahoe, to help with the post-IVF rash. Her fingertips on the pulse in my wrist, she'd shaken her head. "You're not out of the woods yet."

"What do you mean?" I'd panicked.

"Just what I said. This is basically a synthetic pregnancy," she said.

I'd been stunned, too much so to speak. I wanted to swat that word, more hurtful than the *m*-word, from my ear. No matter how they'd been created, no matter how they were birthed, these babies were my flesh and blood. There was nothing fake about it. Right then I knew our time together had come to an end. However, I had yet to fully embrace the alternative to alternative medicine.

"It could even be appointments every day," Dr. Abrams said now.

I folded my arms, tried to look calm.

He continued. "Starting at twenty weeks, you'll be on bed rest between four o'clock and eight o'clock p.m. By bed rest I mean reclining at least forty-five degrees. I can't prove this scientifically, but over the years I've developed this system. For some reason, those are the hours when stuff starts to happen. I want you on this short dose of preemptive bed rest, so you don't end up with the longer version." He said that while, on national average, 50 percent of twins spent some time in the NICU, "our practice has a rate of ninety percent take-home babies." I pictured infants packed like dumplings into white containers.

He sounded proud, and even in the dim-screen brain setting, I could see that 50 percent versus 90 percent was significant. I still felt disconnected. I couldn't absorb that getting through the first twelve weeks was only the beginning, maybe the easy part. Even at birth, there was the coin flip of "take-home babies" and preemies. It sounded like all that stood between us and the NICU was peanut butter.

"That's a lot," I said glumly, eyeing his notes, chucking the crumpled bagel wrapper into the can. Here it was, what I'd feared all along: the medical chute. First there were tests, then surgery, then IVF, then more tests, and finally more surgery.

Dr. Abrams studied my face, and I felt like my teenage self, like I'd done something bad, but also somehow justified.

"This pregnancy is precious. Given your age, and how long you tried, and what it took to get here, you have to look at this as . . ." He paused. "This is it."

I met his gaze, seeing again the tangible human within the doctor. I was glad I'd been picky. All at once, I knew he was right. For the first time, I realized how lucky we were, not just in theory, but with a physical *knowing* of our fortune, which finally filled my body. I was almost forty. I was pregnant after one round of IVF. The odds said I should be online, telling a sadder story in a chat room of compassionate strangers. Nevertheless, in grasping the gift we'd be given, I knew as well how much we stood to lose. Infertility had dashed the assumption that we'd be in a fortunate majority, that our babies would come out healthy and hollering. My friend Linda, a practicing Buddhist, had said once this was the definition of suffering: fear of not having, and then fear of losing.

"We have to take special care," Dr. Abrams concluded. "This pregnancy is a Maserati, and you don't take it to the Ford dealership for care."

Forgetting Buddhism, I loved him for making the pregnancy a fancy car, rather than uttering that worn-out label "high risk" or reminding me I wasn't a late-model vehicle. I loved him for not using the *m*-word.

At home, Ken and I magneted the Abrams Plan to the refrigerator, a good location, considering my bi-hourly visits to the trough. I sucked down eggs, hard-boiled, poached, or scrambled. I also devoured tofu sandwiches with oozing mayo, and anything that would give me a burst of energy, like apples, bagels, cookies. Favorite staples, like *chana masala* and garlic eggplant, had begun to taste funny, though I could still shovel them in. Oatmeal had the right amount of bland, and I stirred in raisins, walnuts, and powdered whey.

I finally waded back into the Internet, to figure out how much one hundred grams of protein actually was—a fuckload, was the answer. More than a handful of walnuts and a slice of hickory-smoked soy, and more black beans and leafy greens than I could possibly consume. The two-egg breakfast didn't cut it, either. It was closer to stuffing one of my smartwater bottles full of hamburger, except I didn't eat meat. I stared into the space over my laptop for a long time, weighing my options.

The next day at noon, I slow-walked to the Middle Eastern place at the top of Solano Avenue. In a nervous voice, I ordered a burger with cheese, well done.

At a corner table, with a fork and knife, trying to keep the patty wrapped in the bun, I mowed it down my gullet, chewing each bite several times. It tasted like something the cow had left on the ground, flavored by the sadness of violating a code I'd lived by for years. I wasn't showing the gods I meant business. There wasn't an ounce of magic, and I didn't feel like a Maserati. I wanted the protein. I wanted my twins to grow. When I finished, I wiped my hands on the napkin, then scrubbed them again at home, then later brushed my teeth twice, flossed, spit, and went back to bed.

Week Nine:

Eating for Three

With my new protein-loading additions of peanut butter, boiled eggs, burnt hamburgers, and trail mix, and now hitting the fifty-two-day mark, my form began its inevitable expansion. My legs stayed like a runner's while my middle rounded into soft paunch, less a smooth melon of elegant pregnancy and more a floppy outcropping of front-loaded muffin top. My breasts got bigger, sore, and hard as Barbie's.

My moods swelled, too, rendering events in Technicolor. I could cry at anything, like the call from Tina where she shrieked with joy to hear my news, just as I hadn't done for her. I welled up at the sweetness of a Citibank ad with two babies, then grew sullen at the thought of more debt. I got irritated with my parents, with parents of singletons, and with anyone who said, "You're having your whole family at once!" as if twins were a tidy shortcut.

Meanwhile, Ken and I were headed to Las Vegas, where he had a physics conference. I would tag along, though I wasn't much of a gambler, unless you counted IVF. Still, as a rickety cab dropped us at a Marriott miles from the Strip, I felt thrilled to get out of the house, to be with Ken and away from doctors. In the Nevada desert heat, I wore old jean shorts and a new maternity top, a ruffled, layered thing that screamed, *I'm pregnant!* as if "showing" in clothes would help me cross the first-trimester minefield.

According to my unexamined logic, vanishing-twin syndrome couldn't happen if they were clearly on display. I sensed the weakness of this solution, but no one had a better suggestion. I'd learned online that in these mysterious cases of disappearance, one twin could absorb his or her deceased sibling in utero. Alternately, the one who perished might remain, becoming flattened into a parchment-like substance, pushed off to the side by the survivor. These revelations were an important reminder: as much as I feared the upheaval of multiples, I yearned for them, too—both, together. That's what I thought about as I crossed the Marriott lobby: *I hope we get a good room, and I hope one baby doesn't ingest the other.*

Other conference attendees—the Europeans with cool eyeglasses, the Japanese in crisply ironed shirts, and the Americans with ponytails and iPods—all dragged roller bags and poster tubes for a three-day science-fest Ken and I called Nano Palooza. Aside from this trickle of physicists, engineers, businessmen, and students, the hotel felt vast and empty, with high, frescoed ceilings and bright Mediterranean tile. At the front desk, we greeted a woman who couldn't have been more than twenty. Rail thin in the floppy maroon polyester uniform, she had a luscious mass of dark curls that framed heavy makeup and slim shoulders. She emanated a sultry boredom, as if she'd rather be in stilettos. Checking us in could have been only her day job.

"We'd love it if you could get us an extremely quiet and private room," I said, a request that sometimes worked. To help the cause, I added, "I am . . . pregnant." For the first time, I claimed it as my own. Ken wasn't pregnant, no matter how much I liked the idea of democratically dispersing the burden with "we." And I was *pregnant*, with the physicality that implied, rather than the more mental "expecting." The word felt visceral, savory.

The zing of satisfaction spread to a stupid grin on my face. Not only could I suddenly own my condition, I could throw it down like a winning card—the pregnancy card! It was Vegas, after all.

Maroon Jacket smiled, raising a plucked brow. "We'll have to get you something special."

Actually, she said nothing.

"Pregnant with twins," I said, doubling down. "Really need my sleep."

A smirk bent her lovely features. "Ma'am, when I get off this job at nine, I'll be dancing around a brass pole. Don't talk to me about sleep."

Of course she didn't say this, either. She only tapped RETURN, RETURN, RETURN with a stiff, manicured finger and, after murmuring congratulations, pushed forward two card keys for room 221—a grim box that overlooked the front awning and parking lot.

"Wow, how could she think this is quiet and private?" I asked Ken, tearing into my backpack for a fistful of granola, dribbling oats down my front.

"We can move if you want." Ken would have stayed in a janitorial closet if it had Wi-Fi, but he'd gotten used to my angling.

"I guess she's like, *Deal with it, bitch. Your life is easy*," which was how I saw myself, in fleeting and increasingly rare moments of clarity. Though I felt uncomfortable, and afraid, my tasks now were simple: to eat, to rest, and to wait. I couldn't say why that felt so strange.

WITHIN AN HOUR WE'D MOVED to the fourth floor, with a view of barren desert and distant high rises. I liked that we could see nightlife in the distance, since we wouldn't see it up close. I'd be in bed by eight—to watch *The Bachelorette*.

Once settled, I studied the room service menu like the Torah. I murmured along to the sacred sounds: *eggs, muffins, potatoes, waffles*. I hadn't had waffles since my parents divorced, when those corrugated Eggo disks, packed with margarine and soaked in syrup, were the sad and thrilling dinner I ate with bare hands. Now they again seemed like an extraordinary treat—outside the normal routine, necessitated by circumstance. Neither could I resist the protein-butter load of a spinach, mushroom, and Swiss cheese omelet. I filled out a room service card for two complete breakfasts.

"How much is that going to cost us?" Ken asked.

"It's a deal, if you count three of us," I explained, patting my mushy abdomen.

I drifted off to sleep just as the sun sank below the blocky-topped cityscape twinkling on the horizon, after setting two apples, a jar of peanut butter, and a plastic knife on the bedside table. I'd be ready for the midnight meal. I thought of the young woman at the desk in her maroon jacket, and what I'd been like in my early twenties: obsessed with freedom, which to me had meant evasion, and adventure.

The last time I'd been in Vegas, Tina and I had been sophomores at the University of Michigan, on a grand road trip. We'd quit our summer jobs in Montana to drive through Washington, Oregon, and California. We worked briefly as migrant berry pickers, lone white girls tearing up our hands and buffing our Spanish among genial if baffled colaborers. Tina, born and boarding-schooled in New England, was a badass woman of the land in her L.L.Bean khakis. She plucked a good haul, impressing everyone. Meanwhile, I proclaimed the joy of working outdoors but often had to nap among the vines, slaughtered by exhaustion.

We then zagged through the Southwest, choosing our route by dangling a needle over an atlas, or always turning right after spotting road kill. We slept in a tiny tent, or dropped in on relatives unannounced. Once in Vegas, we realized we had no cash, so we smoked some pot and slept under the stars in the desert. The coyote skulls and shot-up cans around us didn't matter, or the fact that we'd had only peanut butter for dinner. The point was, we did whatever we wanted, whenever.

After college, when I moved to my aunt Joy's place in the Arkansas hills to chop wood for a winter, Tina came for a long visit. When she got a job farming in New Mexico, I crashed in her tepee. One August, we biked around Alaska, camping in the cool fog of northern forests, roping our food up in bear bags, staring into fires we'd made while declaring ourselves immune to conformity. Tina was unflappable, and I was filled with angst—the perfect yin-yang combination to fuel our escapades. Sometimes two people don't temper each other as much as incite—an unnerving thought as I pondered motherhood with multiples.

Now Tina had twins, and mine were on the way. She had a boy and a girl, stunning toddler redheads, and she'd sent pictures of them, one on her back, one in her arms, my friend in snowshoes in the Vermont woods. Once, stir-crazy in the long winter of their infancy, she'd packed them into her VW bus and driven to Canada. "It was hellish," she admitted, "but worth it."

I prayed that I, too, could keep some part of my twentysomething self, the grit and boldness, that it wouldn't be devoured by the fortysomething twin-mom lady who loved her hotel comforts. As an almost-maybe mother, I also had a fear of vanishing-self syndrome.

Adventure that summer of my pregnancy meant turning off the TV, swallowing a Zantac dry, and trying to sleep on my back. I still ate peanut butter from a spoon, but it was doctor's orders, and I tried to obey. I wanted to stay up late with Ken, take advantage of our time somewhere new, but my body, too, issued direct demands, and all I could do was crash into sleep.

THE NEXT DAY, while Ken mingled with the other physicists in another part of the hotel, I slept in the room, curtains closed. When I woke, I moved my nap to the spa pool, which featured a makeshift waterfall. Fake, cropped, and controlled nature—I would have run from it screaming at age twenty. Now it seemed relaxing, which disturbed me. I couldn't conjure my old outrage.

Later, in search of the food court, I found myself on the threshold of a smoke-filled casino. At rows of slot machines, crystal-headed folks in wheelchairs sucked cigarettes through tracheotomy holes and ashed next to their oxygen tanks. It looked like the waiting room to death, all those people biding time. Once, it would have revved my existential angst. Now, what bothered me most was that they'd poisoned the passage between me and a turkey sandwich.

I turned back to the front desk. Maroon Jacket stared listlessly at her computer, her curly hair perfect. I waited for her to recognize me. She clearly did not.

"Is there another way to get to the food court?"

She shrugged. "I don't actually eat."

Of course she just said "no."

"Are those people really allowed to smoke like that indoors?"

Now she really did shrug. "There's a retirement home across the highway. They come here in the day."

"It's disgusting." I felt twice as bitchy as I'd ever been. "Someone's going to blow up an oxygen tank."

Maroon Jacket looked at me, as if from a distance. All at once, I saw myself, too: almost forty, puffy, hands on hips. Even with twins beneath my ruffled maternity shirt, I surely registered as more pudgy than pregnant, as more impatient than impaired.

"Sorry," she said, without a trace of apology.

I lumbered back to the room and, once calm, called room service for a turkey club. Then I called Tina in Vermont. Within an hour, she'd called me back.

"Missy!"

"Missy May." We used the same nickname back and forth.

"How are those beautiful redheaded twins?"

"Awesome," she said. "Except they always want exactly what the other has."

"True for all of us," I said.

After some more news, I asked, "So, when exactly is the sexy part of twin pregnancy?"

"Uh, what do you mean?"

"Like, when you stop feeling sick, and your bump is cute, and you can stay up late enough to cuddle with your husband?"

"My pregnancy is kinda hazy . . . but, the second trimester?" She didn't sound too sure. "You will stop throwing up."

"I don't have morning sickness," I said brazenly.

"That's sexy right there."

We talked some more. The C-section wasn't bad, she told me, but neither did she remember much. "Can you believe we're both going to have twins? That's so amazing."

It was. We were still on an adventure together, two thousand miles apart.

THAT NIGHT, Ken and I hunkered down to watch *The Bachelorette*. The Marriott had TV screens that gave everyone a wide, stretched appearance, which was fine. I felt larger every day, so why not watch the bikini-clad Bachelorette prancing at twice her girth?

During commercials, Ken and I tapped away on our laptops. Despite Dr. Marion's recommendation to limit pregnancy-related "screen time," we both peeked continuously at sites like BabyCenter.com. It didn't hurt to have weekly updates, constant revision of the kind of fruits, nuts, grains, and legumes the twins resembled.

"Blueberry and Açai have grown into grapes," Ken said.

"Grapes!" I gushed. "Let's call them Green and Purple." Grapes seemed enormous. I could relate to a grape. They were little animals, like Friso.

"They're losing their teeny tails, and those flippers are getting arm-like."

"Their hearts have four chambers," I added, skimming down to the section called "How Your Life's Changing." How *wasn't* my life changing? I read on anyway:

You may feel like an emotional pinball. Mood swings are common now. Try to cut yourself some slack.

The phrase "mood swings" had a link, as if it needed clarification. It was harder to find twin-specific facts and images, but when I did, I stared intently at those cartoon renderings of a woman's abdomen in profile, the pink womb transparent to display its curled passengers. It meant everything to *see* our little grapes.

Meanwhile, on the TV screen, Bachelorette Ali dispensed the ultimate rose for the finale in Tahiti. The place itself seemed incredibly sexy, and all at once I felt old again, and tired, and not sure of our path, no matter how much we'd longed for this day.

I'd recently canceled our own trip to Tahiti—the backup plan Ken and I had made for Christmas should IVF fail. We'd sprung on that extravagant contingency in the weeks of grief following the holidays, when infertility had seemed like cancer, possibly unfixable, and walling us off from ordinary life. If we couldn't have ordinary life, we'd have those sandy shores, the emerald sea. It seemed far enough, and fabulous enough, to block out any hurt. I'd rejected the large hotels there, which "required" attendance at a December 24 "banquet." Instead, we opted for rustic lodging on a more remote island, where we'd make our own salads and slice our own papaya. Despite stunning mountain views, the place was also known for mosquitoes in the air and spiders in the sheets. *Who cares about that?* I'd thought. *Just save me from the Christmas clusterfuck of happy children.* "Book it," I had told the agent, after the insect disclosure. She did.

So, just before Vegas, I'd waited an hour on hold with Air France, saying goodbye to the carefully plotted cliffside Christmas Eve at the least kid-friendly hotel in French Polynesia. Instead, I'd be in the hospital, or at home, recovering from surgery.

I didn't mind not driving aimlessly around with Tina. I didn't mourn Tahiti. I did worry Ken and I would never travel again, at least not anywhere romantic. The thrill of the grapes waned, and I turned slowly to my side.

THE NEXT DAY I DOVE into my book, the best of the tomes about twin pregnancy, according to the good strangers on

Amazon.com. I took it to another pool, read while Don Henley drifted from speakers stashed amid rosemary and cacti.

Mostly, it discussed the importance of weight gain, protein intake, and constant rest, along with the seemingly endless potential complications of a twin pregnancy: gestational diabetes, preeclampsia, preterm labor, premature delivery. It included vignettes of women who didn't follow guidelines and birthed their twins weeks and months early. Their stories of NICU interventions alone were enough to drive me to eat, out of stress, if not obedience. In the section about meals, twin mothers were exhorted to eat right as a form of "empowerment," as one of the few things they could control.

Though I desperately wanted control, I thought this was a stretch. Making myself swallow meat made me feel more helpless than ever. I reached a full-page "centerfold" that diagrammed babies' head sizes at different stages of gestation, to help show the tininess of preemies and the importance of every week inside.

In the realm of twin birth, waiting was the best thing in town.

I flipped to the recipes at the end. Perhaps if I ate exactly according to the expert suggestion, my twins could grow to the ideal head circumference. I sighed at the first few recipes: broccoli quiche, lamb stew. Some days, just nuking water for instant oatmeal seemed exhausting.

Finally, I returned to the room service menu.

Before I made the call, Ken appeared, and the whole point of the trip came back into view: time together. We took a cab to Whole Foods to hit the buffet. I piled vegetables on roast chicken bits, then added a heaping spoonful of macaroni and cheese. I tried to hide the meat from Ken. Though he'd been supportive, for him, my pregnancy diet approached cannibalism. I told myself that for however many months I could, I'd chow down like a bodybuilder. After all, I was growing two brains. We ate overlooking the parking lot, talking about Friso, laughing at ourselves.

"Almost bedtime," I said, though the sun still glinted on the parked cars. "It occurs to me—I'll never be a pole dancer."

"Were you considering it?" Ken asked.

"Probably not," I admitted.

"I'm glad you've come to a decision."

"But if I was, it's too late."

Ken thought this over. "I probably won't win a Nobel. Those guys don't watch *The Bachelorette*."

"But you *could*. My body will change forever."

"We're going to change no matter what," he said.

Then, to cheer me up, "We could stay in Vegas an extra day, do something exciting."

We were both quiet.

"Do you want to?" I asked.

"Nah," Ken said.

"Oh, good!" I clapped. The parking lot glowed in the last desert light. The heat turned to warmth. It wasn't Tahiti, but the feeling of connection had never been as strong, and in our own way, we were far from any place we'd ever been.

Here's what I wish the pregnancy book had told me,

somewhere amid the diagrams and charts: if you can make something easy, do it, because at a certain point, gestating two will be like a road trip with infant twins—hellish, and worth it, too. It will take grit and boldness. Easy is a lovely spot to visit, even linger, though it's not a place to live, and not where love is forged.

Week Ten:

The Pretty One and the Smart One

Back from Las Vegas, I called my mother.

"Still two?" she asked.

"Two what?"

"Two . . . fetuses."

"Oh . . . yes!" I regretted having told her about vanishing-twin syndrome. It had become our greeting, this death check on my pregnancy. "Mom, from now on, let's assume it's two unless I tell you otherwise."

"You aren't at twelve weeks yet, are you?"

"No, but, Mom, I need you to be optimistic."

"I ask because a lot of people have miscarriages."

"I know, but I still need you to be positive. In spite of that."

"Grandma had about five."

This had now become a conversation that required recovery, and we'd barely begun. I wanted her to say, *The worst is over, it's going to be okay, they will be healthy and whole.* Like women everywhere, I was still waiting for a fantasy, a mother-daughter mirage. My particular version entailed less radical honesty and more overt comfort. Of course, the real question was, what kind of mother would I be? I couldn't say those words of comfort to myself. Nor had I come to see even a sliver of what twin pregnancy would teach me—namely, how little of others I could define or control. Not that this would stop me from trying, with the full force of the modern medical universe behind me—or more invasively positioned, to be precise.

The next day, we had an ultrasound scheduled at the perinatologist—part of my "high-risk" roster of doctors. This specialist would tend our kumquat-size offspring as they grew, on board as part of the Abrams Plan—a fairly standard addition, I now knew, for mothers of twins.

Despite my tiredness of all things clinical, I felt desperate to glimpse the babies onscreen. For all my gnashing of teeth over doctor visits, the technology to actually *see* our twins so early on calmed me. We really could look inside my abdomen, like those BabyCenter.com profiles, except they were in 3-D, our actual children. If reality TV acted like a mild tranquilizer, these glimpses of the babies on a black-and-white screen were opium. For many minutes following the procedure, I could escape into an altered world, one in which my worries ceased.

Also, I was excited to go see Dr. Silverman, whom we'd picked, ridiculously, over the other much-recommended guy because of his name, which had the same metalsmithing vibe as ours. It could only be auspicious. He got rave reviews online. Never mind that we'd have to shlep from Berkeley to San Francisco for each visit.

The shiny high-rise loomed in a narrow alley off Van

Ness. Three floors up, the waiting room had clear glass, clean lines, and textile art. My high-risk-pregnancy sisters, perched on boxy chairs, all lived up to the architecture, each dressed for the maternity catwalk. I felt the way I did in Italy, like a boy compared with other women, which was in this case refreshing. One woman wore high-heeled, midcalf boots with eyelet hook closures. I gawked in admiration. As a resident of Berkeley, through some not-quite-conscious process of style osmosis, I wore padded Mary Jane flats, one cut shy of clogs. I would have worn flip-flops, but my feet were too squashed and sore. Just leaning over to fasten the Velcro straps had left me dizzy and tired.

In stretch pants and a big T-shirt, I savored the parade of adorable dresses with black leggings and skinny jeans with clever panels. I understood the urge to give dignity to your pregnant body, though I was striving to do so at Target. I had been to one maternity boutique in San Francisco, called Mom's the Word, for a delirious hormone-fueled spree. I'd felt almost competitive with the one other woman there, who was also my size, but with a singleton pregnancy and her mother in tow. *You've got your mom. Can't I have the last pair of cords?* Still, I'd gotten out with a silk dress for a pending bat mitzvah, "boyfriend cut" jeans I was saving for an unknown occasion, and a pair of stretchy pants I doubted I'd ever wear, so enormous were the legs and waist.

"I feel so suburban," Ken whispered, teasing. "We're going to have to kick it up a notch."

"They should have a shop here, to kill the waiting."

Finally a nurse called us back. After the dreaded pantsless interlude, the tech came and the ultrasound commenced.

In the initial quiet, my first-trimester fears stretched the seconds, as if I were underwater, unable to surface, my chest filled with air.

In a pinched voice, I asked the uniformed woman at the computer, "Still two?"

"Two."

When I heard each heartbeat through the static, I had a flash of peace—the peace I'd been chasing in stores, in naps, in television, in Coconut Bliss, from my mother, from Friso, and from Ken. None of those worked for long, if at all, though calm washed through me in these moments, seeing the babies, hearing each pulse. The waiting ceased. Love stopped time. I let myself arrive.

Even when the tech left, the relief lingered. A few minutes later, in came Dr. Silverman, white-haired and cheerful, an "after" version of Santa Claus, fit and spry. After rechecking our footage on the screen, he spoke with a grin. "Your pregnancy is boring—just what I want."

"We're boring," I chirped.

Ken and I high-fived.

Clothed again, my belly sticky, we returned to the main lobby.

An hour later, Courtney, our assigned genetic counselor, led us to a separate office in a wing behind the front desk. She looked younger than thirty, with blue eyes, black hair, a delicate face, and an asteroid of diamond on her finger. So large was the rock, I couldn't focus on the notebook of genetic disorders, which she flipped through page by page, her hand the perfect twinkling distraction from the scary conversation we were about to have.

When explaining our options for testing, she spoke in a chipper voice, as if to kindergarteners who'd never heard of Mendelian genetics. "For each baby, there are *two* sets of genes," she began.

Ken and I squirmed. We'd already taken a genetic test at the fertility clinic, spitting into inch-long tubes and sending them off at FedEx. I'd used the tricky pseudonym Kathy Gold, lest my saliva turn up something hideous and nullify my health insurance. Now we had a mandatory hour of counseling, and Courtney spoke too slowly, too happily, saying things we already knew or wished we didn't. I wanted our doctors to be upbeat, but our counselors should be able to swear. *This sucks. But this shit is important.*

CVS—chorionic villus sampling—was similar to amniocentesis, except the doctor would extract a snippet of placentas, rather than amniotic fluid. This test also happened earlier in the pregnancy, sometime before fifteen weeks, which meant if we wanted to do something about the results, we weren't as far in—though, in some ways, I felt as if I'd been pregnant for three whole years. By "do something" they meant abortion —CVS tested for trisomy and Down syndrome, among other things. I couldn't imagine the agony of "terminating."

Meanwhile, Courtney stayed delicate in discussing such possibilities, and I wanted to hurry her along. Ken and I were on the same page—a small comfort. We wouldn't go forward with a severe abnormality. So, as Courtney rambled, we slouched in our chairs like middle-aged teens, half tuned out, all but texting in our laps.

"For an extra three or four thousand dollars, we can test for other tragedies lurking in your recessive genes—especially yours, Kathryn. My goodness—Ken's DNA is perfect."

Of course she didn't say that, but the costs of add-ons were staggering, and when we'd done spit tests at the fertility clinic, Ken had passed cleanly, while I had a recessive gene for spinal muscular dystrophy. This, as Dr. Marion had said, was "one of the bad ones."

Courtney flipped through a binder, pointing out the titles and summaries of other rare and hideous maladies, all of which seemed to be named after people, the doctor who first encountered the syndrome or the gene. In addition to the diseases I knew about—risks for us, like Tay-Sachs— there were diseases I'd never heard of. I fixated on maple syrup disease, wondering what horrendous suffering came disguised with the sweet name.

"You might want to tell your sister about the spinal muscular dystrophy gene," Courtney suggested.

Ken and I both laughed, bringing me back to the moment.

My relationship with my sister was volatile, as if the affection and strife between toddlers hadn't aged off but ossified instead. She was less than two years older than I, and we'd been relentlessly compared, divided. Her hair was red and lustrous, mine dull and brown. Karen had always been "the pretty one," while I was "the smart one." To this day, she still squinted at restaurant bills, unable to calculate the tip, while I wasted tons of money in Aveda stores, trying to fix my hair and skin. My future as a computer whiz had been much predicted, while everyone had said that Karen would make a lovely home.

What Courtney didn't know was that having a family

had always been my sister's domain, along with the entire town of Santa Cruz (I got San Francisco, and now Berkeley). Karen liked *Vogue*, I liked *Don Quixote*. She owned citrus fruit, the color orange, girlie skirts. I had broccoli, black, and pants. The list went on, half joke, half the way we saw ourselves.

The problem was, I'd derailed destiny by marrying a great guy and witching up not one but *two* kids, while she continued to date. In our zero-sum sibling system, children were hers. I'd practically stolen them.

On top of the fear of telling Karen I was pregnant, our own identity dynamic was one of the things that scared me with twins. They would always be compared: this one's like this, that one's like that. If I ended up birthing twin sisters, it would be an eerie echo. I had once confessed, as I could only to Karen, a terror of raising girls.

"Really?" she said. "I'm afraid of boys! We can do a swap."

"Why fear boys?" I asked, intrigued that even in gender preference, we'd each drawn a line.

"This is Santa Cruz. They'll smoke pot, skateboard, surf." We were East Coasters at heart. "Why fear girls?"

"I'm afraid they'll be like us," I blurted out, which felt awful to say. "The pretty one. The smart one. Pitted against."

"We had a great childhood," she said, as she always did, though she couldn't remember more than a day or two of it.

"Exactly," I said, rolling my eyes. I was "the angry one."

With all that at stake, I hadn't yet told my sister there were babies on the way. It hadn't gone so perfectly with my parents, and it now made sense with Karen to wait. In this case, waiting meant security. I could put off a painful scene. We'd hold off until the magical twelve-week mark, maybe even until after the CVS. We'd wait for the twin pregnancy to turn a corner, get easier, feel safer.

How did we know we wouldn't have to "terminate"? That wasn't something I planned to share on Facebook. Besides, I didn't expect Karen to be happy for me, not at all. I'd hardly been happy for others when the roles were reversed. So I certainly wasn't going to deliver the twin-pregnancy news and say, "Oh, and if you end up having kids, too, we have this horrible thing called spinal muscular dystrophy."

I couldn't explain any of this to Courtney.

I tersely said, "That's not going to happen."

She paused, then continued her talk. I got the feeling she was obligated, for purposes of billing, perhaps, to fill a whole hour. After a while, I fixated on the CVS procedure itself, which seemed to fall under the bogus Women Can Handle Anything Law. Syringes would draw out the placental tissue samples, which would then be cultured into DNA. Of course, this would happen without drugs.

"So the CVS test itself isn't that bad?" I asked perky Courtney.

"It takes about a minute each, and they give you something to numb the skin."

"But the needles," I said.

"Not that bad," Courtney assured us. "If you did IVF, this is nothing."

I believed her. They would do the test either trans-vaginally or through the outside of the belly. I preferred the latter. My poor seashell was tired of so much medical activity.

On the ride home, Ken stopped and got me an Egg Mit from Noah's, my current favorite: salt, no pepper, no chives, add spinach.

"Are you nervous about this?" he asked, watching me mow bagel into my jaw.

"All I can think about is Maui," I said, through a mouthful of egg. We were headed there in four days, for another physics conference. I knew paradise wasn't a place outside me, but Maui came pretty close.

WEEK ELEVEN:

I AM A BUMP, I AM AN ISLAND

Here's something I learned about twin pregnancy: you can get your money's worth at a breakfast buffet, even in Maui. Ken and I had a week in Makena, where we'd had our honeymoon, four years before, and where, one year after that, we'd begun "trying" to have a baby, when that meant tossing out birth control to launch a carefree and sexy science project. I'd been so confident of quick conception that I'd actually cried—real tears—at the thought of giving up coffee and wine for nine months.

"Coffee isn't a big thing," Ken had said at Ferraro's, over spelt capellini in pesto.

"Easy for you to say!" I sniffled back. "It's how I know I'm *awake*."

I had pounded an espresso after dinner, and we'd sweated out our tension over a raucous game of Ping-Pong in the hotel rec lounge, followed by traditional methods of babymaking back in our room.

The following year, nervousness set in. The "infertility" label had begun to loom, and I would roll my eyes and say,

"I'm not *infertile* because I haven't had a baby *yet*." Not only had I given up coffee and wine, but I'd actively put on weight, at the behest of the Marin acupuncturist. In a few months, I went from 105 pounds to 115.

Year three, I tried to "just relax," which they probably also tell people dismantling bombs. I couldn't unhook the wires of my angst, but I did manage to pray, on the shore of my favorite empty beach.

A year later, those prayers had been answered, but the ache of that time remained, as if scripted into the island's landscape, the way the soft sand had once been sharp seashell and volcanic ash. As newlyweds we'd spoken our vows and mixed our assets, then flown off for some horizontal time. Now, after IVF, we'd mixed our DNA. Our twins were on the way, a different clock ticking now, hard and fast like two tiny hearts.

This would be our last trip to Maui for a while, that elusive chance to "just relax," the narrow sandbar of time between infertility and two babies. Of course, now that I carried twins, *no one* told me to just chill out. Now I had to be vigilant, about protein, water, vitamins, sleep, exercise, and even cheese—it had to be pasteurized, or else.

Our first day in Makena, all that faded away at the breakfast buffet, a buttery-sugar-scented, four-tabled outdoor spread of steel platters, piled with delights sliced, diced, fried, scrambled, poached, dolloped, hashed, and toasted. I could have wept with excitement as I moved in slow motion toward the warm, clean dishes, all of them for us, or so it seemed. We had the place to ourselves, Ken having relented to the 7:00 a.m. arrival. I loaded up my first plate with eggs, rye, scone, banana, strawberries, and melon. I'd never even liked melon—it was Karen food—but it suddenly looked delicious, crisp, and sweet. On a second plate I placed a waffle beneath a wedge of butter, atop a pond of syrup. For round two, I got a pancake and two boxes of Raisin Bran. These I crammed into my beach bag.

"For the night shift," I said to Ken.

"Classy." My gluttony seemed to amuse him. "Don't forget a spoon."

After breakfast we strolled to the beach, then along a narrow, paved road where flowers pulsed with red, pink, and gold, blossoms with spiky petals, delicate stamens, glowing scents. Birds shrieked and chattered, all of it so lush I started to slow down inside, for the first time in months. It was like stepping off some inner treadmill, set too fast, to walk on solid ground.

My legs slowed, too. I'd put on more pounds—five, to be exact—but the load felt like wet cement, heavy and thick. Like many pregnant women, I couldn't stop touching my middle, the mysterious outcropping that hosted two. It brought me to a halt.

"Hey, pokey," Ken teased.

We'd stopped at one of my favorite houses, a sprawling brown shingled affair with views of the sea, where I bent to catch my breath. "Can't we get a cheek swab from whoever's in there? Maybe we're related."

"He's a long-lost relative."

"Who needs a house sitter? *We're* here."

"Who says traveling with twins will be hard? This place is perfect."

This exchange bookmarked the blank page of a different conversation, about our total lack of a plan for taking them anywhere, ever. We'd been blessed with a pregnancy, and we were in Maui. We weren't going to harp on the so-called sacrifice. Not now, anyway. This wasn't denial, nor was it faith. It was something in between, a necessary break.

FOR THE CONFERENCE'S OPENING BANQUET, I could still fit into an old dress—sort of. It strained across the middle, the stomach mush of Las Vegas having solidified into a bump that stuck both outward and sideways.

On the green grass overlooking rocks, beach, and ocean, the physicists and assorted spouses gathered for appetizers and drinks. I loved this crowd, smart but not arrogant, accomplished not only in science but as pilots, pianists, dancers, and entrepreneurs. Before I met Ken, I'd only ever been to writers' conferences, each with varying degrees of heavy drinking, overt despair, and far-fetched flattery. *I so loved your novel about quilting!*

I found the scientists a much mellower bunch. Chatting with Ken's colleagues, I was struck again by how much the infertility years had been a time of not happening, and also not telling. Gatherings like this one had brought jaw-aching anxiety, as I braced myself for the possible questions about our reproductive plans. Over time, even the nonasking had felt strange, anticlimactic, even melancholy.

Yet here we were in Maui, sharing our news of twins. Everyone greeted us with congratulations.

No one asked if we were surprised.

No one asked if multiples ran in the family.

"How far along are you?" Eran, one of the women, asked.

"Twelve weeks," I lied, afraid to say eleven.

No one suggested they might not get born.

Eran's husband, Rupert, ferried me plates full of bread and salmon, all of which I devoured. I thought someone would razz me for no longer being vegetarian, but no one did. It felt exotic at first, to be in a group again and to share the actual events of our life, rather than putting on a good face.

To be myself—an insane, salmon-eating, twin-carrying, dress-stretching pregnant person—was more energizing than any cup of coffee, more dizzying than the best pinot noir.

THE NEXT DAY WE VISITED the calm stretch of ocean that flanked our hotel, and after our mile-long walk up and down the beach, which Ken measured out by pacing, I stripped off my shorts and waded into the waves. I wore a baseball cap pulled low, and an SPF long-sleeved shirt over my bathing suit, aware that pregnancy would change the color of my skin.

Once immersed in the water, I felt lighter than air, as if I could fly. I felt embraced, attuned to an ancient memory of perfect motherlove. The salty taste, the warm-cool feel, the gentle up and down of the waves felt as cleansing as a thorough laugh. Sunlight sparkled on the waves. I splashed, sighed, floated, and flipped. Every bit of physical and mental pain from the IVF receded, a wound clean enough to close at last, and I blended with the deep expanse of blue.

After a while, Ken swam off. "Go ahead and stay. I'll keep an eye on you from the shore."

He watched me from the breaking foam. I waved. He waved back. I felt deeply at home. I didn't need that fancy house by the water, only the water itself. Back in the room, I didn't wash my hair but let it dry salty and hard. I slept on it, inhaling the smell. I swam every day, and it seemed possible there would be moments of respite from the strain of twin pregnancy, the duties, the discomfort, and, above all, the fear of indelible loss.

"Can we stay on Maui until they're born?"

"Sure," Ken said.

I stepped back onto the balcony, listening to the waves sigh, breathing the balmy air. Sleep was heavenly in Hawaii —screen doors, big bed, white sheets. On my side, I could sense the presence of the twins. I could feel them float in peace. For the first time in years, I just relaxed.

AT THE WEEK'S END WE ROLLED through Maui's airport, where uniformed agriculture officials scanned our bags for fruit. I suddenly liked this about Hawaii, despite the extra wait. With air travel, you think the threat is sharp, or explosive, when really it's only an apple, a beetle.

Since we'd put IVF on an airline credit card, we bounced up the totem pole to board the plane early. After a year of waiting without pants, and three years waiting to conceive, it felt glorious to speed through a line—any line.

That day the plane itself felt different. For many years, air travel had seemed like climbing into a death capsule—

only slightly less claustrophobic than an MRI, but roaring over an ocean. Usually I'd be scoping exit doors, checking my life jacket, and downing Valium while Ken shook his head.

This time, I buckled my seat belt, got out my *People*. I didn't have energy to serve as the volunteer air marshal, scanning for the guy trying to ignite his Nike, while also acting as the psychic pilot, buoying the plane with my will. I slumped onto Ken's shoulder. The five-hour flight seemed like an opportunity to sit still, cuddle with Ken, and chomp the pan pizza I'd bought in the terminal food court, delicious even with burnt crust.

Letting go of the fear that we'd never conceive took out other fears, too, like my fear of flying. A whole landmass of dread had shunted off. It took eleven weeks, and a trip to Hawaii, to finally grasp that there were new lives on the way —the babies, of course, but also new lives for me and for Ken. Pregnancy itself wasn't the goal or end point. I could see that clearly in hindsight, like the shoreline as our plane took off. Looking down at the ocean and the break, I felt how much infertility had shaped me, how it had turned me into an island, one I could finally leave behind.

I leaned against Ken until about halfway through the flight, when I staggered to the bathroom and threw up my entire pizza.

"It's nasty in there," I told him, rebuckling my seat belt.

"You okay?" He burrowed around for a barf bag.

"Yeah."

"You think it's morning sickness?"

I'd almost reached the much-vaunted second trimester,

so I barely even considered it. "It's too late for that," I said with a shrug, ignorant with bliss.

WEEK TWELVE:

COMPARED WITH THIS, IVF IS A DANCE PARTY

At Dr. Silverman's, the day of the CVS, a tech named Marcy led us into one of the dim exam rooms. I still had sand in my flip-flops, which made me wistful, and I couldn't move as fast as I had a few days before, which left me worried. Twelve weeks seemed early to slow down. My mouth tasted rotten and minty; I'd thrown up twice the night before and then rebrushed my teeth each time. I still didn't believe it could be morning sickness, not at this late date. Supposedly, that kind of symptom disappeared around this time in pregnancy—no way it could be emerging.

Ken helped hoist me onto the chair, and I attributed my queasiness to my body's anticipation of the CVS. My stomach burbled a mild warning. Otherwise, I felt strangely relaxed.

As Marcy zipped the scanner over my belly, I noted that the bump had hardened even more, expanding its arc into a defined dome. We watched the screen as she located the babies—still two!

"They look like yams," I whispered.

"Yam A and Yam B," Ken said.

Marcy tapped notes on the computer. *Parents insufferable*, or whatever they record.

"You can empty your bladder a little," she said, arranging the gear on a metal tray—long needles, plastic tubes, and belly goo in a clear condiment bottle.

My eyes skittered over these tools. Had it been an interrogation, I would have spilled the beans at that moment. I blocked them out as I wrapped the huge paper towel over my butt to get to the adjoining bathroom. My pants were off, as usual, even though Dr. Silverman would likely "go in" through the belly. The nurse on the phone had instructed me to drink a liter of water upon waking and hold it until I arrived. This way, my full bladder would press the babies farther into view. IVF had taught me it didn't take that much to fill the tank, so I'd just chugged on the way to San Francisco. On the dwindling menu of twin pregnancy's small pleasures, mild defiance was one of the most delicious.

CVS had a risk of miscarriage, but we'd heard Dr. Silverman had never had an incident. Apparently it mattered who did the procedure, but wasn't that an unspoken fact with anything medical? The more doctors I saw, the less I thought of them as a uniform crowd. They were frighteningly mortal, but some had turned themselves into superathletes, the Kenyan runners of medicine.

I still was not terribly nervous. Maybe Hawaii had dazzled me into long-lasting calm. Maybe I was shallow in my keenness to know whether we had boys or girls, to start picturing them as real, as turning into humans, rather than complications, or at least human complications. I'd recently handled a pair of red sparkly shoes, handed down from my friend Grace, wondering if I was wrong to fear girls. Oh, the girlie things we would do! Then I had put them away. In the end, CVS was a buffer against regret. If we didn't do the test, and one or both babies were born with something awful, we'd always look back and kick ourselves. Of course, twins made the stakes more than twice as high. One sick child, we could perhaps tend—but what about the other? What about two? It was better to take the needles.

When Dr. Silverman didn't appear for twenty minutes, then thirty, I started to wiggle. My bladder now felt ready to burst.

"I would rather be poked than wait to be poked," I said to Ken when Marcy left the room.

"I know," he said, gently poking me behind my ear.

I laughed. "It's not funny. Let's leave."

"Okay."

Of course we didn't move, Godot without pants.

Then Dr. Silverman bustled in, cheerful and sage, all in white, his beard like Papa Smurf's. For a moment I relaxed again. Even as he was about to plunge needles into my uterus and suck out bits of placenta, he acted like a guy heading out with friends.

He commanded the ultrasound station, whirring the gizmo over my bump in fast swirling motions. "Okay, yes, we'll go through the outside." He was agreeing with himself, which was always good.

Great, I thought, relieved.

Marcy loaded the needles.

I moaned. "My bladder has to be full, right?"

Dr. Silverman startled. "We're not doing it to make you uncomfortable."

It would have surprised him, I thought, to know that a year earlier, I had considered most medical doctors overpaid sadists. Now, in the upside-down world of twin pregnancy, they were more like saviors.

"You ready?" he asked.

"Yes."

"It's important that you don't grab at the needles."

It was my turn to startle. "Of course not."

The shot of Novocain stung, delivered by an enormous hypodermic, not the dainty little needles Ken used for IVF. My spine arched. The lights dimmed. The show was just getting started.

I don't want to report CVS as a horror story, but I would like to be honest. For the full Vagina Lady version, read on. Otherwise, skip to the last paragraph.

The props department had overdone it with the CVS needle, borrowed from a low-budget alien-abduction flick. A clear container stuck off the syringe part, which I supposed would contain the extracted matter. With a regular Sharpie, Dr. Silverman carefully pen-marked two spots on the bump, one high and to the left, one lower, toward my pelvis. I peered over the achy hilltop of my belly. He put an index finger on the first target and plunged the needle in.

I gasped.

It felt exactly like a giant needle being plunged into my uterus.

A pulling-sucking sensation followed, the squirming

movement of stuff coming out—bits of placenta. I crushed both of Ken's hands in my own. It was all I could do not to swat the needle away. It went on and on. In this case, the poke was much worse than the wait. A couple times I muttered, "Oh, *fuck*," and then, "Sorry" when the first was done.

"No problem," Marcy said. "We hear it all. That's actually polite, relatively."

Here's the thing about twin pregnancy: someone plunged a needle into my uterus, and I got through it. Then they loaded up and did it *again*.

For the second time, I grabbed the top of the seat behind me, then Ken's hands.

Again Marcy and Dr. Silverman huddled over me. Apparently, Baby B was harder to reach and took some maneuvering. The minutes splattered open into something else—quivering, undead road kill. "Oh, *fuck*" didn't even come close.

They spoke in hushed tones. More tissue wriggled out of me. It was the farthest from nature I'd ever been. Deep, deep in the wilds of medicine.

When it was done, Dr. Silverman lifted the vials, as if in a toast. They were full of chunky, foamy white matter.

"These are good samples," he declared, upbeat as ever.

He showed us the name labels for us to confirm. KATHRYN GOLDBERG. I barely knew who I was, but I nodded just the same. Sounded familiar. Many people might have filled the void of my mind at that moment—my husband, Tina, our doctors, our babies—but instead I focused on the incoming image of Courtney, our genetic counselor, who'd assured us CVS would be minor compared with fertility injections. All I could think was, *Holy fuck, has that woman ever talked to someone who's done IVF?* The CVS was nothing, and I mean *nothing*, like that.

As I dressed with trembling hands, I was stunned but not upset. It was like stepping out of crumpled metal after a car accident and feeling elated to breathe. When the numbness of shock gave way, I felt almost ecstatic. It was done. And soon we could peek at their genes. Surely, some sacrifice had been necessary to behold such mystery.

At home, on bed rest for the next three days, I fell like timber onto our sofa. I wasn't supposed to move, lest the body's recent trauma trigger a miscarriage. I couldn't imagine doing anything else. I passed hours stroking Friso, eating Szechuan eggplant, regurgitating Szechuan eggplant. I stared at the red rug, the sunlight, shadows, dust. Friso licked my face.

I kept replaying the needles in my head. For some reason it made me laugh, in that way that laughter creeps in on inappropriate occasions, like how I laughed on the way to my grandfather's funeral, because my nose had so much snot. Sometimes the awfulness of the body is funny, the way it likes to remind you how little you control.

After watching the blue bruises that splotched my abdomen, I called Linda to report, and to boast.

"That's, like, Civil War–type stuff," she said.

I realized something new. "The primitive and the cutting edge now intersect."

I felt proud. Accepting turned out to be harder than doing, even if the multiples book said that eating hamburgers and taking naps would make me less helpless. Maybe I'd never "get used" to this, but endurance, it turned out, bestowed power.

It took a week to ten days to hear the outcome of CVS. For once, I felt okay with the wait.

Week Thirteen:

The Art of Barfing

The moment should have been perfect. We'd gathered in the basement rec room, just as I'd envisioned during that time-killing, room-cleaning, feng shui frenzy before surgery and IVF. Our friends Mark and Ali were over for brunch, along with their dog and two young children, all of them mingling happily with Friso. While Ken toasted bagels upstairs, I settled onto the red couch that had arrived with the "you're pregnant" call from Dr. Marion. A mere nine weeks later, I felt huge, tired, and clearly pregnant.

"We are so happy for you," Ali said, from her perch on the enormous ottoman.

I sipped a cup of fresh carrot juice from the juicer once meant to cure my infertility. It tasted sweet, like victory. My gut rumbled. I opened my mouth to express my own happiness but instead vomited orange mush onto a decorative pillow and the hardwood floor.

The silence of our guests echoed against my retching.

"Sorry," I croaked, standing up, catching bile with my hands.

"Oh God, don't be!" our friends said.

Ken ran in with a trash can, too late. Then he went for towels. The rec room had been christened, but not the way I'd hoped.

As much as I wanted to stay and bask in our revived social life, instead I staggered back upstairs to bed, dizzy and spent. Wrapped around the five-foot, tube-shaped pillow Ken had named Longfellow, I realized how little I'd anticipated the realities of twin pregnancy. If I had pictured anything, it was Ken rubbing my feet while I emanated a "pregnancy glow," burnished by our second-honeymoon intimacy. I'd be busy folding organic onesies, comparing swatches from Restoration Hardware, or making friends in prenatal yoga classes. In the mornings, the stork would flap by with double bags of cash. The flip side of the paranoia that had begun with infertility—fear of never having children, the feeling of being cursed—turned out to be delusional optimism.

Certainly, I hadn't included round-the-clock morning sickness in my vision, and I hadn't even known about "round ligament pain." "Round ligaments" sounded like something Friso would chew on, harvested from buffalo and renamed to disguise, the way dog-treat bull penises were called "bully sticks." It hardly described the agonized stretching of innards, not to mention skin, as the bump expanded daily. I hadn't pondered sore breasts, sleeplessness, or weird red welts on my neck and jaw.

I now understood that pregnancy would not be perfect, nor perhaps even fun. Still, it would have been nice to get through a brunch.

THE MONDAY AFTER THE carrot juice incident, we headed to San Francisco to see Dr. Jennifer Young, part of the Dr. Abrams Dream Team. Each start and stop in the Bay Bridge traffic jarred my insides. I grasped at the bump, grumbling, "Ouch!" and, "Not so fast!" Once we parked on busy California Street, my stomach gurgled so loudly it blotted out Terry Gross. Ken sprinted into Walgreens, only to return breathless, with bad news. "They've banned plastic bags!"

I leaned out the passenger-side door and chundered on the curb.

Ken rubbed my back. "I'm so sorry."

"*I'm* sorry," I said.

"Don't *you* be sorry," he said back.

"That was my one safe meal," I whimpered. "Poached eggs."

"I can see that."

I hoped Dr. Young would have something good to say, some magic remedy, as I slunk foul-mouthed and miserable into the office. In the waiting room, Ken handed me a magazine called *Fit Pregnancy*. On the cover, a grinning woman wore skinny jeans and flashed her toned arms from a sleeveless blouse. Her hair had been combed, and her bump looked like a small pillow.

I batted the magazine. "Is she even *pregnant?*"

Ken chuckled, put the glossy away.

I wasn't done. "Put some vomit on her chin. Then maybe I'll read that."

"Yolk chunks in her hair," he added.

"I want to read *Having a Fit, Pregnant*."

"*Pregnant Hissy Fit*."

Maligning the cheerful publication passed that day's wait. Even into the evening, we dreamed up our own magazine.

"I have a better name," I told Ken, as we shuffled through our numerous remote controls for the evening's TV.

"Let's hear it."

"*It's Twins, Bitch.*"

"That puts the onus on others."

"Exactly! Who *wouldn't* want to read that?"

In the meantime, I wrote a new list, "The Rules of Barfing." I read them to Ken:

The Rules of Barfing

1. Be prepared.
   Carry a plastic bag.

2. Avoid toilets.
   They stink, they're hard to clean, and the lid can bonk your nose.

3. Use a small plastic trash can, which is portable.
   Can be combined with the plastic bag.

4. Accept the nausea.
   This too shall *not* pass—until you throw up.

5. Trust no food.
   Favorites can turn on you at any time.

Ken listened generously, as if I were penning an interesting equation on his office whiteboard. "Do those barfing rules apply to life?"

"Be prepared, be paranoid, accept it's going to suck?"

"Rules for warfare," he said.

"Or dealing with family," I said, thinking back on the last few days.

When I had told my mother I'd been barfing, she had said, "Doesn't it make you feel bad for Karen?"

"Why would I feel bad for Karen?" I asked, shooting from zero to hostile in seconds, as seemed to happen more often in my hormone-soaked state.

"The allergy attacks," my mother said. As a child, my sister had suffered days-long bouts of vomiting. I'd forgotten: Karen owned throwing up.

"No, I do not feel bad for Karen," I said. "That was thirty years ago."

"That kind of sickness always makes me feel bad for Karen."

"I feel bad for *myself*," I said, in the tone of voice that left me most daunted about my readiness to be a parent, especially to same-age siblings.

My mother didn't seem to notice. "Have you *told* Karen, by the way?"

"No, I have not."

It was time. A secret in our family lasted about as long as a Popsicle in East Coast August. Once, my mother in Bethesda told my uncle in San Diego something so soon after the confidence that, given the cross-country time change, he knew about it *before* it even happened. The only reason no one had leaked to Karen so far was a generalized fear of her reaction. We all knew kids were "hers." *Accept that it might suck.* I had told my father and Belinda, and they had cheered. How much more could I expect?

"I'm going to tell her soon," I said, feeling queasier than

I'd been all week. I took a Zantac, but my heart still burned. I desperately wanted someone to *get it*, and my mother was the stand-in for all the people who didn't. Which was nearly everyone.

Before I went to sleep, Ken brought me my special trash can, set by the bed. He straightened Longfellow, tucked me in, kissed my cheek. He held Friso over my face to do the same.

I looked up at Ken and the panting puppy, and there it was, in the reflection of love in their faces: my moment of perfection in a twin pregnancy.

Even later that night, when I leaned out over the mattress to cough up that evening's oatmeal, I found one comforting thought amid the pain and mess of the nausea: I didn't need a doctor's test to know the babies were on board.

Week Fourteen:

Counting all Chromosomes

We crossed the river under cover of night, out of the first trimester and into the second. Though weary, we were at least on the right side of the statistics for miscarriage: the chances that our children would get born had much improved, even if my "morning sickness" had not. I crossed off days on a calendar, as if filling the white numbered squares could box up time and get rid of it, like junk from the basement. The weird spike in patience from the CVS experience—which helped me through an entire week of waiting for results—had started to wane.

The report supposedly rolled in after seven days, and we'd reached eight. Late news could not be good news. I feared Courtney had a map of our chromosomal tragedy in a folder on her desk, but was too busy sampling champagne fountains and burnishing her engagement diamond to call.

"What if . . . ?" I asked Ken.

"Don't say it. Don't speak the words."

"But . . ."

"The thing to remember is the outcome already exists."

The call came Saturday afternoon. Curled in bed with Longfellow between my legs, I stared into our yard, untended all summer: the long yellow grass, the thick fireplace ivy, a massive flowering jasmine. It billowed over a fence and up toward our window, as if it might poke a tendril inside to also hear this news.

Ken rushed in with the phone, put it on speaker, and dove beneath the covers. "You ready?"

"God, yes."

"Everything looks great." Courtney sounded perky as ever, and I immediately forgave her for misrepresenting the CVS. "Do you want to know the sexes?"

"Yes!"

"Do you want to guess?"

We clutched the phone between us.

"Kathryn?" Ken said, as if it were the mother's right.

"Boy . . . and girl?" I said.

"Two boys," Courtney said.

"Wow," I said. I'd had a feeling, because of the red sparkly shoes, and those elephant and stegosaurus hats, but it seemed like cheating to say it after the fact. I did anyway. "I thought it might be two boys!"

Ken hung up, and we fumbled to embrace, my arms flailing. It took a full minute to roll onto my other side.

"Hi, boys," Ken called down to the bump.

"We can't wait to meet you!"

"We are going to talk tonight about the Giants."

"Do you want to name them Tim and Brian?" I knew the pitchers' names.

We were having two boys, a thought big enough to wipe out other worries. Having grown up in a girl world with my mother and sister, I thought boys were a mystery. Maybe they'd be as polarized as my sister and I, but it wouldn't be over hair. They wouldn't play the cruel games of attack and withhold—in my mind they'd just hit, which I'd discourage with clever modern phrases like "Use your words!" Two boys meant a cleaner slate; I could mess them up in fresh and original ways. Above all, it felt joyful to know something so tangible, so absolute. I would have gushed over the word "daughters" just as much, or marveled at one of each, but now the fantasies could take focus. We would have two sons.

Later that day, Ken and I sat in our sunny kitchen, with the phone on speaker again. I reminded myself to keep my expectations low, follow the rules of barfing as they pertained to family: be prepared, limit the mess.

We dialed Karen's number in silence.

This time, after a brief round of hellos, I spoke. "So, we have some news. . . . I'm pregnant. And it's twins."

"Oh my God!"

I held the phone back. She hadn't been told. When Karen lied, her jaw locked so tight it was audible even on the phone, upbeat speech squeezing through the clench. Now, she sounded truly unhinged.

"Congratulations! Twins!" She seemed more excited receiving this news than I'd been at the fertility clinic—not a trace of ambivalence.

"Thank you." I reached for an apple from the fruit bowl, exhaling. Ken gave me a thumbs-up across the table.

"That is so great. I am so excited."

"Thank you," I said again, not ready to be done. "Can you believe . . . twins?"

"Oh, everyone has twins."

"I guess." I wondered whom she meant—celebrities, maybe. Technically, we twin moms were about 3 percent of the population, though twin births increased year over year. As of 2011, one in thirty babies born in the United States was a twin, and, less scientifically, it did seem as if everyone knew at least one person who had them.

"Do you know if it's boys or girls?"

"Two boys." I stroked the bump, my sons.

"You always wanted boys," she said.

I felt sheepish. "I would have been happy either way."

"My neighbor has twins, and they are the cutest."

"I so appreciate your excitement."

"What's not to be excited about? I can't wait to be an aunt!"

"I wish I'd told you earlier. We've been waiting for results of an amnio-type test." This was sort of true. Secrecy was my terrain. Blurting was hers.

She gushed a while longer, said she'd make the drive to Berkeley in the next two weeks. I kept myself from saying, *So you're not mad?*

"I have to come up soon. My sister is pregnant with twins!" She shouted this, and I realized she must be on her balcony. "Is it okay I told my neighbor?"

"Sure," I said. Karen was the public one.

"I assume you don't want me to put this on Facebook."

"Maybe not yet."

"Mom and Dad know?"

"I just told them."

"Hmmph." The competition was there, but not with me. "You told them *first?*"

"Barely anyone knows. I still have to tell Aunt Joy and Uncle Bob, the rest of the extended family."

Instead, that afternoon Karen let it slip to Joy over voice mail. Then my mother, who heard that Karen had leaked to Joy, told the rest of my uncles and aunts. "I had to," she explained, "for 'political reasons.'"

Did the boys in my belly also belong to others? It seemed, for the first time, that they did. There were aunts and grandmas and great-uncles also getting born. The tribe would get two babies at once, without the trials of twin pregnancy—*that* was a good deal. I sent out e-mails with news that wasn't new, or even only mine.

Week Fifteen:

Shit People Say to Women Pregnant with Twins

Despite the excitement of the CVS results and the relief of telling my sister, the fatigue and nausea dampened everything like a persistent rain. The two seemed to fuel each other—exhaustion after throwing up, tired stomach heaving lunch. I huddled indoors while July rolled in with shiny sun and dry heat. Laughter and smoke from our neighbors' barbecues wafted through our screens. I wanted to be out there, wearing a tank top and drinking lemonade, but mostly I felt too sick. I wondered when the side effects would move to the side and leave me to focus on the pure celebration of this pregnancy.

Speaking of celebration, we had an array of family events on Ken's side, for which I'd splurged on that silk high-waisted dress in the San Francisco maternity shop. The morning of my niece's bat mitzvah, I found myself trapped in the garment's upper reaches, arms flailing overhead, as if to signal drowning, the dress jammed above my double-wide bump. When I finally popped my head through the neck hole, panting and astonished, I tugged the skirt down.

Breathless, I confronted the mirror. The mound strained the clever pleats. The frock that had hung so sweetly a mere month earlier now looked like a failed effort at watermelon smuggling.

I'd planned to wear that dress to the end. Now I saw it wouldn't even go to breakfast. I wiggled it off. All that money and hope, the stupid competition with the other, barely pregnant singleton mom at Mom's the Word, and I should have let her have it. I sank to the bed's edge, sapped, clad only in maternity leggings, Bellaband, and sports bra. All that bulletproof gear to hold stuff in, and I still felt like coming apart.

"Am I huge?" I asked, when Ken came in from his shower.

He looked at me to see whether I was kidding, heading for a meltdown, or both. I wasn't sure myself. He wore a towel, his beard freshly shaved. His body looked streamlined and mobile. I marveled at his ease of movement, as he bent to his clean-laundry midden to find boxers. I knew he was delaying an answer, wisely.

"My dresses don't fit." I rose, turned sideways in the mirror. "I don't even fit in the mirror's frame!"

"That, you can control. But you've definitely had a growth spurt," he said finally.

"That's good, right?"

"It's great."

"It feels weird." Not only was my body not my own, its inhabitants outnumbered me. I joined Ken at his pile, pulled out a pair of his old sweats. "Do you mind if I wear these to temple?"

"Not at all." They had holes in the knees and one thigh. I could have slipped into a garbage bag and gotten the same response.

After hanger whacking through my closest, I resigned myself to a paisley maternity hand-me-down with a giant bow. Thus gift-wrapped, having stashed tamari almonds and a Scharffen Berger bar in my purse, we headed out. The weekend-long affair launched with a service Friday evening, followed by a Torah reading Saturday morning, with a post-script reception early afternoon, culminating in a party Saturday night. I thought I could do it all, minus the Friday night, which I'd missed because I'd been horking into a Target bag.

For the morning service, we would get up in front of the congregation and sing a portion of prayer. Ken had practiced for hours, while I'd glanced at the sheet and listened to him sing. From our bench in the front row, we faced four car-peted stairs, which we would soon have to climb. Our niece read beautifully and with confidence, and I watched with admiration tinted only by my fear that I would crumple or trip on my way to the podium. How terrible would it be for the massive pregnant aunt to fall in the middle of the bat mitzvah? The dress bow would unravel as I slid from Ken's grasp, my be-Spanxed legs flashing the *oooohing* crowd as I tumbled. The rabbi would say something somber and reas-suring as the medics carted me away.

Instead, when the moment came, I clung to one of Ken's elbows, while his mother clung to the other, and we climbed together. No one fell. Most of us chanted our portion of the song quietly, in mumbles, while Ken belted out the Hebrew like Bruce Springsteen, a sound that steadied me as much as his arm. I did not throw up—another prayer granted.

BACK AT HOME, between the service and the party, I sobbed tired tears but still dragged myself out to the evening reception. Having told my sister, and with my own large Jewish family now on board with the twin news, I remembered anew the importance of these collective rites: the equivalent of a subscription to worthiness, to love itself. To miss even one event put your membership at risk. Having two babies on the way made it seem more important than ever to affirm the sacred ties, to show that we belonged, and, at the end of it, to partake in the much-touted fudge fountain.

So I swayed in my now-wrinkled paisley, pestering the caterers about the buffet and gazing glassy-eyed at the tween revelers. The seventh graders danced while the DJ egged them on. There's nothing like watching thirteen-year-olds dance to make you feel old and enormous.

"We are having two boys," I told one cousin, trying to rev myself into gear. I'd been daydreaming of boys, thinking about Ken singing his heart out at the service, hoping our sons would be just like him.

"Too bad you didn't get one girl. It's so fun to dress them." She, of course, had a boy and a girl, two years apart. She flapped a hand in dismissal. "Doesn't matter—with twins you won't leave the house for a year."

I had no idea how to respond. Only a week out of first-trimester miscarriage conversations, I recognized the gender comment as a huge upgrade, and also that the strange things people had to say about my pregnancy had just begun. It wasn't only my family of origin dishing out the weirdness. The comment about never leaving the house poked a raw nerve—I shared that fear myself, unable to picture any normal activities with two babies in tow. I tried to calm myself down and ended up in a bathroom stall. I forgot about holding it together. I needed metal walls to keep it all out.

After a while, I snuck outside to the parking lot, settling in a corner that overlooked a golden field flanked by eucalyptus. A Mossad-looking guy came close, then left, having established I was a morose pregnant lady, not a threat.

Finally, I called Tina.

"Oh, that shit doesn't stop when they're born," she told me. "I'm still stunned how many people say, right in front of my kids, 'I'm sure glad *I* don't have twins.'"

"What do you say?"

"I say, 'Me, too.'"

Tina also said this, which would stick with me for a long time: "Try to remember, everyone's reaction to your pregnancy is really about themselves."

I wished I weren't so sensitive, but my emotional skin was like the skin on my belly—thinner by the day. I'd stayed for this party out of a sense of tribal obligation, surely lost on my young, dancing niece, as well it should have been. I did make it back for the fudge fountain, a burbling volcano of chocolate, though I couldn't even lift an arm to dunk a piece of fruit or bread.

This was before I would learn one of the better lessons of twin pregnancy: you're allowed to say no. This rule was the corollary to the harder rule: you have to say no. My duty was no longer to the family around me, but to the one within.

By the end of the week, I wrote a new list:

Crazy Shit People Say
When You're Pregnant with Twins

1. "Do twins run in your family?"

   This question generally meant, "Did you do IVF?" In what world is that not personal? You are going through the most invasive medical odyssey of your life and don't need invasive questions to top it off.

2. "Do everything you want to do now, before they come."

   Should you be skydiving, or perhaps bungee jumping? You can hardly "do everything you want to do" while also living in fear of eating the wrong cheese.

3. "Get lots of sleep—you'll never sleep again."

   This isn't insider knowledge about newborns.

4. "The first year is hell."

   Hell is also the people who don't *get it*.

5. "You're having an instant family!"

   Though this is often meant to be positive, who says two children make you a "family"? Family are the people who love you through any outcome.

6. "A woman I know had twins born early, three pounds each. She had to move into an apartment by the hospital so she could breastfeed them in between their surgeries."

If you have a friend diagnosed with cancer, you don't tell them the story about your aunt Nell, who died after months of chemotherapy. You tell them about the aunt who went through cancer and still rides her bike to the farmers' market at age seventy.

Things You Should Say
to a Woman Pregnant with Twins

1. "Congratulations!"

   That word, or that word embellished with a few other upbeat sprinklings, like "It's going to be amazing" or "Your child will have a sibling to play with!"

2. "You look great!"

   This doesn't have to be true. It helps.

Week Sixteen:

Mobster Meets Twin Pregnancy

I couldn't remember why we'd signed up for anything at 10:00 a.m. on Saturdays, much less Advanced Obedience for Puppies, except the sense that having two new babies and a rambunctious TUD was going to be difficult. Somehow, we pinpointed *the dog* as the hard part. The rest, we could surely figure out: double breastfeeding, sleep training, diaper changing. We'd always been fretters and planners, yet we envisioned a blurry postnatal world in which the babies by their own instincts would nurse, nap, and nuzzle, while those soiled Pampers carted themselves off to Yucca Mountain. In recent prepregnancy physics trips to Japan and Italy, we had carried every guidebook, gadget, and map we could find, crammed into massive suitcases, along with shoes for every contingency and backup coffee gear. Now, we were moving to a foreign country—parenthood—and acting as if all we'd need was extra underwear and a few Clif bars. We'd ask directions from the natives when we got there. As I mentioned earlier, extreme paranoia has a fraternal twin: delusional optimism.

Despite this, I wasn't sure Friso was ready for "advanced" anything, and certainly not "obedience," though he did frequently go outside to poo. He'd also mastered a few tricks from Puppy Basics. He would turn for his name, lower his hindquarters for "sit," and gallop our way for "come"—all with speed and enthusiasm, as long as we shook a bag of peanut butter treats. Otherwise, he twitched his nose and clicked across the floor, just barely compliant. Sometimes, faced with a stern command but no edible incentive, he actually yawned in response.

In the class, in a rec building at a local park, I needed two chairs, one for my butt, and one for my feet. Ken, in his uniform of black T-shirt and jeans, did all the dog-related drills. Sprawled there at the sidelines, feeling queasy and cumbersome, I remembered my own jeans–black shirt days. Now I wore a stretchy fuchsia dress from Target, the most appealing feature of which had been its $7 price tag— cheaper than a burrito on Solano Avenue. Beneath this, I wore a beige "brace," intended to help secure the bump but in fact an itchy and distracting bandage that gave my midsection a barrel-ish outline.

While Ken forced Friso to focus, I let my mind wander.

That morning, I'd tried to read one of the books Dr. Marion had recommended, *The Girlfriends' Guide to Pregnancy*. I had found it useful—as an object to hurl across the room. The author's chatty voice struck all the right notes for a pregnant woman, just not me, with two babies taking over what I'd always considered "my body." I wanted to join the "sorority" she described, but I felt too afraid and too big. I would not fit through their doorway. I'd packed on fifteen pounds already—a number the "girlfriends" considered excessive even at full term.

Now, about halfway through puppy class, a crunching sound of Velcro brought me back to the moment, as the bump brace began to crack open. Overheated and constrained, I realized why Friso so hated his harness. The indignity!

Friso, meanwhile, had abandoned his task of walking from one spot to the next and ignoring a treat in the middle. Instead, he sprinted off course, slid into the instructor's feet, and flung himself over for a belly rub.

Ken and I made eye contact, sharing a silent laugh.

"He gets so distracted," Ken said, as we leashed him up at the end of the hour, after a brief chase, Ken running, me shouting, "Stay!"

When Friso refused to walk, Ken cradled him, legs curled, head nestled, our dog looking much like a newborn human, white fur suit aside.

"Speaking of distracted, should we maybe take . . . a baby class?" I said suddenly.

Both of our mothers had suggested this, but we'd rejected the idea, tartly informing them that those seminars had nothing for twin parents.

Ken thought it over as we reached the car and Friso squirmed away from his crate. "Didn't you order some books?"

"Only that one I threw this morning."

"If you find one you like, underline the good stuff."

At least we were on the same page: the denial page.

AFTER CLASS WE DROVE two blocks to Chester's, which had outdoor seating, and the waiter brought Friso a bowl of water while Ken and I devoured tofu scrambles. Then Ken swooped into Love at First Bite for a chocolate–peanut butter cupcake, removing the icing cap for me, the way I liked it, and taking the bottom for himself. A stranger had once observed this arrangement and said, "You must still be newlyweds."

The sweet peanut butter icing tasted so good, with Friso at my feet, I thought, *I need treats, too.* I knew what they were: TV time with Ken, wantonly cruising the Internet, clicking things into the cart at Giggle.com, slurping down bowls of Coconut Bliss. I'd settled for such petty pleasures, such easy escapes, when I knew I'd be better off busy or, at the very least, exercising, meditating, *preparing.* How did you prepare for two babies? Maybe I wasn't up for a "baby class," but we should at least have IKEA parts strewn on the floor around us as we built cribs and tables. Somehow I couldn't find the discipline, even on the days I didn't throw up. Like Friso, I craved rewards without the work. I had made myself the pregnancy equivalent of a TUD.

As I licked the icing from my fingers, I gave myself the task of getting to the pool, thereby retroactively earning my cupcake top. At home, I knew I'd better get dressed in the bedroom, lest I crap out on a bench in the chlorine-scented changing room. I gathered up my towel, slathered on sunblock, and stuffed myself into my maternity bathing suit. Still sugar-high from the icing, I found courage for a long gander in the mirror. My legs had remained much the same, as had my arms, while my midsection looked glaringly pregnant, only much further along than sixteen weeks, and much wider across the middle. In some way I preferred my appearance in fitted swimwear to the weird tentiness of clothes—maybe that's why celebrities liked to strip down when pregnant, though I hadn't seen any of the famous twin moms (Angelina, Julia, J. Lo), at least not in the hallowed pages of *People*. That magazine, unlike others, I didn't need to throw.

I couldn't decide what to put on over my swimsuit. I settled on a white cotton robe, another maternity hand-me-down, and went to say goodbye to Ken. He'd camped out on the TV-room sofa to watch the Giants.

"You're going in *that?*" he asked.

"What?"

"All Vincent Gigante mafioso in your robe?"

Apparently I did have a famous-person look-alike: the mobster who'd tried to feign insanity by puttering around New York in terry-cloth sleepwear.

"I'm not faking crazy," I explained. "This is the real deal."

At the pool, I chugged through the locker room. Maybe I'd throw up and appall everyone, but I would do so in the act of nurturing my babies and myself. That had to count as preparation. Outside, I shucked off my robe and lowered myself into the aqua box, into the one lane clearly marked SLOW. The only other swimmer, an elderly woman with a pink floral swim cap, drifted upstream with a barely detectable sidestroke.

The water felt cold, nothing like Maui but also

wonderful, the way it lifted me from my aching feet. I began my own super-slow-mo breaststroke, head and baseball cap carefully aloft. My lane mate and I drifted back and forth for about twenty minutes, until a goggled swimmer in a tight black suit flapped into our peaceful sea. She zoomed down the middle of the lane to pass us, splashing us both with her speedy freestyle.

The next time she plowed by, I didn't budge, and neither did the woman in the rubber cap. The three of us faced off in an intense confrontation of lap-swim chicken.

The freestyler got caught in a logjam and caved; same again on her next rounds. Finally she rose to her feet and squinted. Then she ducked beneath the rope and was gone. The other woman and I flashed smiles. *Don't mess with the old and the pregnant. We're the slow-lane Mafia.* We were on the same page: the crazy page.

AT HOME, I felt clean inside, and I soaped up in a hot shower, dribbling coconut oil on the bump. In pajamas by 4:00 p.m., I wrapped up in the white robe again, liking how it felt, a cloak of protective madness.

While the sound of cheering baseball fans drifted from the man cave, I unfolded myself downward to sit cross-legged on the bedroom floor. I would meditate, as I hadn't done in ages, not since before IVF. I hadn't wanted to face my mind any more than I'd wanted to face my body, but now I'd make the day a twofer. Perhaps I could even bask in the pleasure of this, that we'd gotten pregnant, that we had two —two!—babies on the way.

I let my hands flop backward on my knees. In the stillness, I could feel the tickling inside, kicking. It had been going on for days, gathering force—the boys swimming in their own underwater dance. I liked to think they'd woken up in temple the week before, moved by Ken's loud, proud prayer.

Meanwhile, Friso decided my rhythmic breathing and closed eyelids meant it was time to attack. His paws hit my shoulder, then my neck, before he leaped onto my lap. I stayed still. He yapped twice.

"Shhh," I whispered. "Mommy's meditating."

He pushed against me, sniffing.

"Shhh," I said again.

Down the hall, Ken shouted at his team. "Yes! *Yes! Go!*"

Friso licked my mouth.

It tasted like kibble, but I held my ground.

"Kathryn, Kathryn, the Giants are crushing it!" Ken shouted. "You gotta come here! Come!"

I sighed, gave up. I headed to the TV room, Friso trailing.

Ken rewound the screen to show me a fresh home run. While Pablo "The Panda" Sandoval rounded third, I sank down onto the sofa, and Friso hopped up, too, his tail wagging wildly at the mood of the room.

Mediation could wait. Friso was insane, and so was I— insane even to try.

As I stretched out with Ken, gathering pillows for the bump, I thought how it had become popular to say, "The definition of insanity is doing the same things over and over and expecting different results." But didn't we as human beings do the same things over and over all the time, in order to change? It was what we'd done in canine obedience school. Didn't all the hard and worthwhile things take repetition, commitment, and blindness to results? Wasn't that how exercise worked? Wasn't that how love itself functioned, in the slow, day-to-day tending?

This sofa moment *was* the meditation—babies stirring, dog resting, husband rejoicing. Friso, finally content, wedged himself on top of both of our legs. He taught us what the books never could, his puppy priorities the ones we needed, too: determination, togetherness, unstinting love. Dog class aside, he trained us.

WEEK SEVENTEEN:

TWIN PREGNANCY IS "TORTURE"

"Dr. Silverman is on vacation. You'll see Dr. Meanie today," the woman at the front desk told us.

Perhaps I should have protested, but I'd just finished throwing up in the parking garage and didn't feel like opening my mouth again.

Once on the exam table, leggings shucked aside, I stayed quiet through the initial scan. After a few pleasantries with Marcy, our now-familiar tech, I couldn't help but perk up at the sight of the babies on the screen. In addition to the ultrasound monitor, a second TV hung in an upper corner, so I could easily watch the black-and-white shots of babies inside me. They had clear faces, eyes closed in giant heads, hands tucked beneath chins, legs folded to belly. I knew from my friend the Internet they could now grimace, like their mom.

"I'll make a disc for you," Marcy said when she'd finished. "Dr. Meanie will be with you shortly."

Yeah, right.

The doctor did come, and I barely registered her presence in the dim room, a woman with a white coat, straight reddish hair, and an air of cranky haste, as if she'd missed the last Muni bus and we were drunken bums waiting at the stop.

With brusque greetings, no eye contact, and a few taps on the computer screen, she gave her verdict on our unborn children. "They look fine."

"Fine?" I missed Dr. Silverman's effusive cheer.

"Fine," she repeated.

"Fine is one notch away from fair, which is one notch from poor. In surveys."

Ken chuckled. The doctor did not.

"Do they look *good*?" he translated.

She nodded, swiping the goo off my belly, as if she'd boarded the bus now and my skin were the sticky seat. "You might want to consider a fetal echocardiogram."

Panic hit, a slap to my face. "Is there a problem with their hearts?"

"No. But heart defects are more common in babies from IVF, and all defects are more common with twins."

Suddenly I missed Courtney, with her gentle, singsong tone.

Meanie and Ken launched a rapid back-and-forth about percentages and the odds of heart abnormalities—a duel of scientists, escalating into math. Apparently it was 0.15 percent more common for IVF babies to have some kind of heart problem, whereas the general population had a 0.5 percent chance.

"So it's just over point-one percent more likely than half a percent?" Ken asked.

I lay there like an overturned turtle, miserable and helpless. As far as I could tell, twins made everything twice as likely.

Meanie seemed to agree with Ken, who said, "Hmmph."

I reached for his hand, gave it a *let's go* squeeze. "Can you hand me my pants?"

Ken asked one more question. "Kathryn is constantly sick in the car. What can we do?"

Meanie shook her head. "Nothing. Twin pregnancy is torture. Get used to it." Then she left.

We were struck silent. Those were the actual words.

"Wow," Ken said finally.

"Torture?" I said.

"Get *used* to it?" Ken asked.

"*Seriously.*"

"I don't want to do that echocardiogram, do you?"

"No," I said, relieved and excited that we felt the same way. I assumed Ken would want the data. We shared a moment of wicked resistance, as if the rudeness of Meanie's manner canceled out the point of her suggestion. It was easier to be mad at one person than at a host of symptoms, to dislike a doctor instead of your own body, especially with precious twins inside.

"TORTURE? TORTURE? Should she really be saying that?" I ranted over my *bibimbap* at the nearby Korean deli, squirting hot sauce on the rice, as if into Meanie's eye.

"That was so weird," Ken said.

"Let's make sure not to see her again."

"She's like a cold Midwesterner." Ken, a native of California, had this impression of midcountry.

"What's torture are people like her," I said.

In a weird way, she lit me up, righteous indignation stoking the furnace. *I* could say it was torture, an exclusive prerogative of twin-moms-to-be. Doctors, on the other hand, should stay calm and positive, let the patients dabble in wrath and dread. Otherwise, the entire system broke down. Wasn't that partly why they dealt with cadavers in medical school, to learn to stifle certain honest reactions? They had all the power, they wore the pants—but we alone, the naked patients, had the right to bare our feelings.

At home, after Ken headed to the lab, I googled "twin pregnancy," then skimmed past all the official sites, like BabyCenter.com and MayoClinic.org, looking for the personal. I didn't need the soothing and bland. Those sites were a gateway drug, a legitimate way to close a work document and ease into the emotional fringes of the Internet, the territory Dr. Marion and Dr. Young advised against. I knew it would be a circus of opinion and myth, the place I now belonged. Finally, I refined my search to "twin pregnancy sucks," rather than "torture," refusing to dignify Dr. Meanie's remark. Three blogs popped up.

These were my sisters, my sorority, those who knew the initiations of IVF, heartburn, and ambivalence. I was supposed to be overjoyed at "having my whole family at once," and my gratitude for that wish granted knew no bounds—at least in theory. That didn't stop me from needing my physical misery reflected in a secret communion online. Here, total strangers spewed details about intercourse with "dh" (darling husband), excesses of "cm" (cervical mucus), and problems with "bm" (poop). The oversharing didn't matter to me. What I really sought was unbridled complaining. I didn't savor anyone else's suffering but needed to know I wasn't alone. That Ken and I had worked so hard to make these babies left me guilty that I lacked bottomless bliss.

Also, in the midst of reading about other twin moms' rashes, nausea, aches, and stitched-up cervixes, I sometimes stumbled on practical solutions to the endless discomfort. One woman swore that sleeping in a papasan chair helped her heartburn and allowed her to rest. *See, Dr. Meanie, maybe you don't have the solution, but Pier 1 sure does!* I called Ken at work.

"I think I can fix the nausea with a papasan chair," I told him, breathless.

"One of those satellite-dish seats?"

"Yes. I can sleep propped up. I *know* it will help."

"I'll be home early to go with you."

By the end of the day, we'd brought one home, lashed to the roof of Ken's Nissan.

Friso adored the white faux-fur cushion, as did I. At night, I garnished it with six more pillows, one between my legs, one beneath my head, one beneath the bump, and the other three as props or to seal the cracks. I brought my iPad, the trash can, my phone, a full bottle of smartwater, and a spare comforter. I still felt nauseated, but so far, dinner stayed down. At least we tried, no matter what Meanie said.

Ken came to tuck me into the bamboo nest, to say good night to the boys and me.

"They're kicking a lot," he said, his hand on my belly.
"They're okay," I said. "I feel it. Their hearts are okay."
Still, I knew we'd end up doing that test.

WEEK EIGHTEEN:

TWINS AND THE RELIABLY WILD

A few weeks after I told her the twin news, my sister, Karen, drove up from Santa Cruz for her first visit in many months. Despite her living only two hours away, in recent years we'd rarely spoken face-to-face, relying on the masks of phone calls and e-mails. Whenever people said, 'So-and-so is like a sister to me,' I wondered which part they meant. The ugly fights? The stupid competition? The long silences?

The year I had married Ken, my sister and her fiancé had broken up. She'd cried at my wedding, and it hadn't seemed to be with joy. I didn't blame her in the least. From childhood on, it was like we had the emotional version of the syndrome that can strike fetal twins, those who share an amniotic sac. One feeds off the blood of the other, and both get sick. That's how it felt with Karen and me, like we'd grown up believing there wasn't enough, so anyone's gain was the other's loss—except it left us both worse for wear.

Since that time when I got hitched and she got single, the pettiest of topics could spiral into a waltz through the minefield. Once, when I'd failed to inquire about her nap, as in, "How was your nap?" we exploded into shouting, then didn't speak for months. I constantly let her down, in ways large and small.

Despite all this, on a cool September day in my eighteenth week, with two boys roiling in the bump, boredom and discomfort so dominated my mind that nothing marred my excitement to see her. Even a fight would trump the monotony of twin-pregnancy fatigue. Besides, I vowed to avoid conflict. Pelé and Beckham could hear now, and we needed to set an example.

I put on one of my new Target maxi dresses, a blue muumuu with ruching beneath my rock-solid breasts. Soon after, Karen appeared at the door, wearing a bright cycling shirt and brown cargo pants. She carried with her a backpack, a water bottle, and a sticker-covered MacBook, since any visit included her popping onto Facebook. Her bobbed red-blond hair shot out in every direction, probably from an early-morning mountain-bike ride. I knew visiting me qualified as "backstage" for her—no need to dress up. I'd crammed my own tangles into a ponytail. Everywhere was backstage for me.

She glanced briefly at my sheepish smile, gawked at my bump. "Oh my God!"

"I know," I said. "It's crazy."

"You look great!"

It wasn't true, but I loved it nonetheless.

"I miss being the guy," I said, one of our jokes, and she laughed. For years, she'd shown up everywhere in short flowery dresses, while I wore Haberman shorts, multipocket camp shorts that she said looked like our elementary school gym teacher, Mr. Haberman.

"I'm the guy now," she teased.

"Yeah, right."

With a *clickety-clack* on the wood floor, Friso joined us, saving us. Karen dropped down to play with him, obediently rubbing his belly as he sprawled on his back. When Friso felt good, it somehow transferred to me, dog-person kinship at its best. I got mushy watching him with my sister, who generally disliked animals. Friso was a love vector, our safe vehicle of affection.

"Let me show you the papasan chair!" By phone I'd shared the details of the Pier 1 excursion, along with endless accounts of heartburn and throw-up. If we sweated the small things, we also bonded in the banal. No one could show more enthusiasm for a bamboo chair than Karen—another singular fact of sisterhood.

"I totally want to see this." She followed me to the bedroom. "Would you consider selling it to me when you're done?"

"Sure. We could *give* it to you."

"I could use more seating for parties." Karen regularly had fifty or sixty people over on Saturday nights for cake, dancing, chats until sunrise.

I couldn't remember the last time we'd had a party bigger than my friend Linda. Even before pregnancy, I'd moved toward tameness. I didn't know if my former adventure self would ever return, especially as certain stodgy traits emerged, ones that shocked me. I cared deeply about shoes being put away, dishes whisked from the sink, and tables cleared of junk. These were fixations I'd detested in both my mother and my father, though I now often nagged Ken to pick up this or that. I couldn't quite believe having two boys would make the house neater, or me more relaxed. I thought about Tina and me, twenty years earlier, driving willy-nilly through the American West, and wondered how I'd feel if our kids did the same. Not mellow, I decided. I'd mocked my parents for wishing I'd pursue a stable career but suddenly found myself saying to Ken, "With twins, you get one doctor *and* one lawyer!" Of course I was joking—or was I?

Perhaps someday my sons would turn to Karen, as I had turned to my mother's sister, Joy, the free spirit, the sub-verter, the one who had hitchhiked around India barefoot, lived in a tepee in Montana, grown pot with her husband, Merlin, in the Ozarks. For years, more than either of my parents, I'd sought her for advice, for acceptance, and a place to crash in my flailing twenties.

Watching my sister check her phone and fire off a text message, I felt decrepit. I couldn't type with my thumbs, and I'd only recently learned what "hashtag" meant. I grew older still as Karen helped me move armloads of clothes out of the nursery closet and into our bedroom. Like an elderly person, I saved up chores for able-bodied visitors.

After a while we drove two blocks to Nature's Express, my once-athletic self reduced to breathlessness after a few steps. Seated outside, shaded from the sun, we talked about her boyfriend, whom she knew to be temporary. I felt the unfaded ache of her broken engagement, her earned reluct-ance to trust anew, and my own sense of survivor's guilt.

Then she reeled off parts of her hectic schedule: biking

at Wilder Ranch with a bunch of guys, processing photos from her China trip, teaching classes in social media. "Next week I'll be in Yosemite."

The only solid plan on my horizon, beyond more doctors' appointments, was my firm intention to take a shower.

I put down my avocado-kale wrap, unable to swallow the weirdness of my immobility. Just getting to Solano Avenue felt like a journey. Our recent trip to Pier 1 had been an escapade. Of course I'd be more active after the twins were born, but it wouldn't include Yosemite or China. Even a neighborhood stroll would entail wrangling two babies and myriad gear. It wasn't that I longed to travel—I'd had my fill and more—but I worried again about who I would become, that I'd turn dull and small, no fire for my boys.

Karen spoke breezily of her freedom. She hadn't pursued it, as I once had. In some ways it had been foisted upon her. Nevertheless, it enveloped her, bestowed a spirit of fun that I knew our kids would love. If I'd "stolen" children, she was living part of "my" life, too. I'd always thought I would be the "rebel aunt," or at least reliably wild.

Please, God, don't let me do this to the boys.

With twins, there would always be comparisons: the big one and the small one, the shy one and the talker. Even if Ken and I refrained, the world at large likely would not. Somehow, I'd have to let this go.

It all seemed overwhelming, until my sister lifted a tissue-wrapped square from the paper bag, the last bit of our order. My vision zoomed to the cubic inch of a walnut brownie.

"You didn't." My appetite returned.

"I did."

"I'm drooling."

"I'll cut it in half," which she did, carefully, with a plastic knife. When you've divided everything over a lifetime, you learn to slice fair, especially when it comes to dessert. Besides, no one of us could ever claim chocolate as our own. Like sisterhood, it was so familiar, so intense, we kept coming back. We each ate one side of the brownie, and it was more than enough.

"You're going to be a great aunt," I said.

"I can't wait." Karen sounded upbeat.

"They're going to be yours, too." Maybe with the boys, we could keep the sharing clean.

"I know."

"Friso misses you," I said to my sister, the closest I could come to *I miss you, too*. Back at the house, we both stroked him for a while, and then she headed home.

Week Nineteen:

Vagina Monologue for Twin Pregnancy

There should be a Vagina Monologue from the moms-to-be of twins. *Hey, leave me alone. Is it still today? Ugh. Seriously, I don't care if you need another ultrasound. I don't want to see anything with a condom on it unless it's attached to my husband. Unless it's brandished for recreation. No, not tonight, though. Already showered. Closed for business.*

My own transformation to Vagina Lady was nearly complete, eerily speedy, the way the babies now had ears and eyes and practiced their World Cup kicks all day. I had grown obsessed with my pregnancy experience. By now I not only marked my calendar to note passing days but also broke down each day into clustered hours. This hardly eased the wait, but I couldn't resist trying to *quantify* my experience and thereby manage discomfort. As a kid I'd negotiated with my parents for a precise quota of peas—*I'll eat seven*—because parsing and counting each pea subtracted flavor. If I counted time, I could focus less on its content. *Do everything you want to do right now*, said the tireless advice-givers. What

I wanted was to lie on my side without aching, retching, or crying. What I wanted was a break from the doctors.

"What if we assumed everything was fine and didn't go at all?" I asked Ken.

"Then it would be 1970."

"Why can't they make better technology, so it's not always me without pants? Like those airport scanners, only safe."

"Then it's 2070."

Unfortunately for my vagina, I was scheduled for a "fetal survey" with Dr. Silverman. By ultrasound they would take detailed measurements of both babies, officially Baby A and Baby B. Presumably, this would be another way to find defects in the head, limbs, spine, brain, and assorted organs.

Tina, who rarely complained about anything, recalled this as "the longest ultrasound ever." Her twins were eight months old now, and while her pregnancy had been a blur, this stood out, she said.

"How long will it take?" I had asked the front desk at Dr. Silverman's when we'd scheduled the appointment. All of my own defects were on open display: fear, reluctance, impatience.

"About three hours," the receptionist said, clicking her mouse.

How could anyone tolerate a three-hour ultrasound? I found even brief incursions excruciating. I wondered whether I could do this without Valium. Would I risk a drug-induced birth defect to scan for other defects? I could sneak a sedative, and it would likely be fine, except for the fact that I would bask in worry and self-blame forever after. I decided I would not. Somehow I'd get through.

ON SATURDAY I DRAGGED myself to a prenatal yoga class at Seventh Heaven, paying $14 to the pierced woman behind the desk. I still believed yoga to be its own kind of sedative, though I'd mostly done self-styled, homeschool stretches, downward dog, and modified warrior. Going to this class after years of avoidance was like showing up in the emergency room of awareness practice, so a Hindu SWAT team of flexible yogis could transfuse me with calm.

First, I had to empty my bladder. Of course all the other pregnant women were also gathered in the bathroom, as if by a watering hole on the African savanna. I spotted a woman with a belly so tremendous, it visibly trembled beneath her stretched T-shirt. She could barely get her hands to the sink. I figured she would go directly from class to Alta Bates hospital to deliver. Lucky her, so close to being finished. Or maybe she was an earth mother who had begun labor but stayed relaxed enough to make a pot of quinoa and go to yoga before sauntering to the family bed to push. My theories aside, I had to admit she seemed strangely vacant, with rings beneath her eyes. The gray of her skin, the mass of her bump —she looked like an extra in some postapocalyptic film.

When class started, I learned that she was pregnant with twins.

Not only that, she was a mere ten weeks ahead of me, nowhere near delivery. Nor was she keen to chat about my twin-pregnancy second-trimester hopes and fears.

"I'm about to do the fetal survey this week. I'm a little worried about the duration of that ultrasound," I told her, restrained, I thought, for not babbling about vagina fatigue.

"Huh," she said, declining eye contact. No need for Valium there.

I could tell how different from the singleton moms she looked. How different *we* looked. Their bumps didn't squeeze out sideways or jut so far forward. Mine dangled over my yoga pants at an awkward angle, with an asymmetrical jaunt to the left. Both babies were currently transverse. Hers was just behemoth.

"You need to be really careful," the instructor told me, as if I weren't moving at the speed of geology.

Every pose involved blankets and blocks, and I felt impatient with each setup to stretch, as if every three minutes I had to tear down my awesome sand castle. Once in a pose, I felt impatient with that, too. There I was, waiting again—waiting to feel better, waiting to give up, waiting to go home.

"Breathe in and connect with your baby," the instructor said, and I remembered that in yoga, most often I was breathing in and connecting with my bad attitude. I knew it was petty, but I resented that she said "baby" in the singular, since some of us were carrying two.

"This stretch is excellent preparation for birth."

"I'm having a C-section," I announced proudly.

Actually I froze, retreating into my twin-pregnancy bubble. Rather than arch my upper back in cat pose, I curled on my side on the mat while the boys pedaled their legs, as if they had the energy I'd lost. I sensed the instructor standing over me, and I didn't care. Amazingly, I plunged right into a half nap, worth $14 itself. Thus, I dispelled a partial unit of the morning.

At the end, I watched the other twin mom creep to her car in the parking lot, gawking at her shape in a way I would soon come to loathe, when it came my turn. All I thought that day was, *Will that be my fate? Impossible. She must have an undetected triplet.*

I called Tina at home, and soon after she e-mailed me a picture of her belly before birth. I immediately clicked the message box shut. *Nope, not for me, no thank you.* I had only to get through the next clump of four-hour sets, and then the fetal survey, after which Ken and I would go out for *bibimbap*, unless I was in a stress-induced coma or a strait-jacket.

"IT'S ALL EXTERNAL," our tech, Marcy, assured me, the day of the fetal survey.

"Oh," I said, slumping in relief.

"You thought this was a three-hour vaginal ultrasound? I'm amazed you showed up," she said.

"You don't even know."

In the end, the ultrasound took a measly ninety minutes —faster, and also easier, than the prenatal yoga class. The goo and transponder zipping on my belly shocked my pained navel, but not much more. I asked Ken to count backward from one hundred, in increments of seven. We passed the time by emptying it of meaning. The babies' limbs and bones and organs measured fine.

Without even meaning to, I breathed in, connecting to my sons.

Week Twenty:

The Pantheon of Badass Twin Moms

A few months before I met Ken, I went on a Caribbean cruise with my father's family. While Belinda's four kids plus spouses partied in their multiroom suite in the ship's bow, Karen and I divided our cramped cabin with a love seat between our two cots. Like all shoddy borders, this one didn't separate so much as delineate the positions from which we could snipe. By morning of the first day, we barely spoke, though she talked about me, on the phone, as if I weren't a few feet away. "Kath is being *silent* because she needs *space* to write in her *journal*." With my mug in one hand and pen in the other, I inked complaints about Karen while she broadcast hers about me. We'd boarded with pure intentions, but the high seas uncorked something else, as if the maritime laws governing our relationship were looser, harsher, and more prone to punishment.

After a week, surrounded by open ocean, a hostile sister, and indifferent stepsiblings, I considered attending the ship's meeting for Friends of Bill—the cruise newsletter's sly code for Alcoholics Anonymous—to my mind, a gathering devoted to compassion and acceptance. I longed for the company of a group where I could speak my feelings. A makeshift family of addicts sounded perfect. So many of my favorite authors had been there: Augusten Burroughs, Anne Lamott, Mary Carr. It seemed they'd made AA friends who took their calls in the middle of the night, friends who filled their lives with wisdom, laughter, and God. Maybe I was an alcoholic. I'd been guzzling wine since the first day on board, the morning of which Karen had given me the double middle finger before dawn, for "flushing the toilet too loudly."

Years later, now pregnant with twins, I found a group to which I legitimately belonged—the local twins club—and which every twin mother recommended (I continuously stopped them on the street). Unlike my vision of AA, I feared Twins by the Bay, more comfortable with the role of possible addict than mom of two. I imagined the new and expectant parents' meeting would be like one of those self-help cults where you couldn't leave the room, even to pee, unless you vowed to breastfeed both babies until their bar mitzvahs. I figured a Bay Area twin parents' group would be packed with earth mothers.

I couldn't say what exactly defined an earth mother, but she wouldn't have wept at giving up coffee or mourned outgrowing jeans. She wouldn't waste hours reading reviews of diaper bags on Nordstrom.com. Instead, she would focus on things like how to actually care for her infants once they were born. From my vantage point of inferiority, everyone else seemed smug.

Meanwhile, the sofa mother ran intermittently in my bloodline—the tired, supine, exasperated mom with a forearm flung over her eyes. My grandma Charlotte, in this pose on the couch, used to lament not having aborted my aunt Joy—in my aunt Joy's presence. As an adult, Joy had fled Chevy Chase for a yurt in Arkansas. My own mother had escaped only down the road, to Bethesda. She tended Charlotte through numerous surgeries, after which my grandmother would open her eyes in the hospital bed and say, "Leslie, if the cancer doesn't kill me, those shorts you're wearing will."

Despite her not-so-warm-and-fuzzy upbringing, my mother had been a super stay-at-home mom to my sister and me right up until the divorce. She'd been Girl Scout leader, cookie baker, homework helper, and carpool driver. Though she liked to sleep in, she'd been queen of crafts. We made our own dolls, afternoons that involved yarn, cornhusks, and hot glue. When my father left, my mother, too, had a period of prostration, perhaps shocked into horizontal recovery, mostly in bed. It was brief but striking—even the least sofa-prone women can be struck flat. When she returned to grad school and then to work, we shifted to an empty-refrigerator, every-girl-for-herself roommate situation, complete with disapproval of each other's boyfriends and fights about the sink.

Now, decades later and for the first time, I felt compassion and understanding for my mother and grandmother both. As the living room sofa cushions left a faint waffle print on my cheek, a great ancestral sigh welled up inside me. Down to my tired bones, I knew what it meant to feel overwhelmed.

And my kids weren't even born yet.

In my magical-medical thinking, maybe this was why I kept throwing up—self-disgust. This was what drove me to the Twins by the Bay meeting, despite my pariah parent feelings: the loneliness of the sensation that I had once again prefailed, expressed most precisely as morning sickness. *Desperation is salvation*, the AA sponsor part of me said. *Get help.*

All this stirred in my gut as I waddled into the lobby of Bananas, a bland, boxy 1970s building off the freeway in Oakland.

"Is this the Twins by the Bay new and expectant parents' meeting?" I asked a distracted woman behind a computer and a counter, in my mousiest voice.

"Upstairs," she said. "Elevator's that way." She took a second glance at me, one with more surprise. Only a week before, I'd given that same twice-over to the spacey twin mom at the yoga studio, to my now-retroactive regret. *It's twins. I'm pregnant, not blind.*

On the second floor of this "family center," I plodded down a hallway filled with the faint musk of diaper. Kids' books, old car seats, and a rickety stroller lined the hallway, which, in my hormonal state, seemed ominous and sad. It was as far as one could get from, say, enjoying a glass of sauvignon blanc on a sunny day by a field of lavender in Sonoma. This was fluorescent lights, Desitin waft, and baby shrieks. I sensed that a majority of humans in the building did not use a toilet. *If the pregnancy doesn't kill me, this place will.*

In a room at the end, beyond a circle of chairs, three women hunched over pillows and blankets. They were all topless, laughing, and chatty. Below them, tiny pink vampires splayed on their backs, gorging themselves at their mothers' breasts. Two of the women with pillows propped their babies under each arm, in a double football hold. The other was on all fours, dangling herself into her twins' mouths, her own head turned to the side in conversation. I pegged her immediately: the homeschooling, bootie-knitting, wood toy–only, militant earth mother. If I ever turned to formula, she'd be out there, burning a bottle in our front yard.

My sister would have sauntered up, said hello, taken names. Here were the twin moms I'd been looking for everywhere!

A moment later, I was sobbing in a bathroom stall.

This wasn't what I had pictured when Dr. Marion had mentioned "the risk of twins." I had thought only of the medical hazards, not so much the destruction of all things I enjoyed. I didn't want this life unfolding in a building called Bananas. I wanted to be outside running, in a café with writer friends, or having tons of sex with my husband, like Katherine Heigl in *Knocked Up*. I hadn't asked for twins. Okay, maybe I had, a little, putting in two embryos and then praying fervently to keep them both. But I hadn't known it would be so stark. I hadn't known I'd feel so sick, cranky, and downtrodden. I hadn't pictured myself leaving the club of fellow artist introverts to join the most exhausted moms on Earth, those too put-upon to wear shirts. Now I'd finally done it. I'd joined *a support group*, and not a cool one packed with fabulous, post-partying quirky characters who spoke in endless witticisms. It was one where we'd discuss sore bottoms, cracked nipples, and high forceps. It was a congress of Vagina Ladies.

In my stall, I unfurled toilet paper, blew my nose. I debated going home and left a message on Karen's cell phone. Even without reaching her, I knew what she'd say. *You always recoil from groups. You're afraid of being judged.*

To prove her wrong, I flushed the toilet as loudly as I could and left the bathroom with tissue in my fist.

To my horror, seven or eight more women were clustered out there in the hallway, talking and excited. They bent over each other's massive strollers, reciting names and ages: "Graham and Ethan, four weeks," or "Ada and Riley, sixteen weeks adjusted." The newest babies looked like pale prunes, the frailest like old people shrunken to five pounds. The bigger ones had pumpkin heads atop Carter's pajamas and two-tooth grins. Most women pushed their progeny in a horrific device I'd recently learned about, which everyone called a "double snap," a rickety metal frame that held two car seats front to back. Had they heard me crying in there? Rant-whispering to Karen's voice mail? If so, they were kind enough to leave me alone.

I patted myself down for car keys, envisioning my getaway. I'd have to stand there anyway, jamming my thumb on the elevator down button. I realized my sister was right. The group struck me as the basic unit of judgment, like a jury. Like a family.

Yet I couldn't deny that these women seemed pretty focused on the wrangling of strollers and babies, and not on my puffy-eyed suffering.

Somehow, I fell in line with the twin-mom herd, let them sweep me back down the hall. Tentatively, I took a chair in the circle. The three women who'd been breastfeeding were now shirted, cooing over their babies.

More women trickled in, until there were about fifteen of us—and also two men—and of course babies in sets, like Noah's Ark. Three of us were pregnant. I stared at them the way Friso gazed at other small white dogs we passed, nervous and alert, curious but ready to bolt.

One of the pregnant women was tall and thin—except for the basketball bump—in loose pants and a T-shirt. She sat with crossed legs, which I could no longer do. During introductions, she said she was a single mom of one, and a lesbian, who had conceived twins in a bid for a second child. "I don't know how I'll handle three. And my entire community is like, 'What were you thinking?'"

I calmed down one degree, forced into sudden perspective. I certainly wasn't alone in my fear, and if people expected me to be doubly happy or twice as doomed, no one had questioned my right to have two babies. Not even grudgingly, I saw I had things to appreciate, not the least of which was a partner.

The woman continued, "People are like, 'You need a network.' Where should I get that, Target?"

Her snarkiness was soothing, too.

The other pregnant woman was oddly lithe for thirty weeks along and sounded cheerful, despite being unable to drive anymore, having passed out twice behind the wheel. A full eleven weeks behind her, I could have crushed her dainty frame. She looked like a pregnant Angelina Jolie, whereas I'd morphed into the large purple figure from the McDonald's playground.

"I'm wondering if anyone can recommend a pediatrician," she said, worried, of course, about her babies—not an earth mother in this concern, I realized, just a normal person.

My eyes burned as the introductions reached me.

I choked my name out before the inevitable waterworks. "I feel so overwhelmed. I throw up all the time, and I'm . . . overwhelmed." I couldn't get more out.

The room felt still. All eyes turned to me, but it was the opposite of a group's collective critique. Cars whooshed outside. Babies cooed. I blew my nose. It was the first minute in memory that I didn't want to replace with the next minute. Kindness hummed in the depth of that quiet.

One of the moderators spoke up. "Start with the nausea. Don't be afraid to ask for the drugs."

"Do whatever you need to feel better."

"It does usually pass, but it still sucks."

For the first time since I'd learned I was pregnant with twins, I felt a glimmer of being understood. Even my most loving singleton-parent friends didn't grasp my anxiety, and their advice sometimes came as oppressive, whether about breastfeeding, cosleeping, or training a baby to pee over the toilet. Briefly, I felt reprieve from the shame of not being blissful.

At a glance, most of the women were older, some single, several gay, some fancy, some casual. I wondered how many of us had done IVF, though I knew that in this rare safe zone, no one would ask. We'd all endured the stupid comments, and we practiced prison code: you don't ask what anyone did to get here. We were all innocent. People had been through stuff.

The sympathy kept coming.

"It is harder than a singleton pregnancy."

"It gets easier the minute they're born."

The two men were silent helpers. One had come with his wife and baby daughters, who slept like little champs in their car seats. The other was a granddad, lying fully on his side with his grandbabies. Later, he wandered around holding extra kids, bouncing them to quiet.

The discussion moved to air travel. The woman who'd been breastfeeding on all fours handed out TSA regulations for all the moms so we'd know our rights (it turned out she was a high-powered attorney, not an earth mother ringleader). She talked about pumping on the airplane.

"You go in that little bathroom?" someone asked.

"Oh, no, I pumped in my seat, with a blanket. I travel for business a lot."

"What about the other people in your aisle?"

"I ask them if they have kids. That helps."

I decided she was a badass.

Then the topic shifted to sleep training—whatever that was. I'd recently heard a twin dad on NPR mentioning sleep in increments of minutes and had willfully blurred the rest of his tale. Now, I watched the group's lone granddad tenderly make gaga faces, until I grew distracted by the woman next to me. She held one baby in her arms while rocking the other in a car seat with her foot. I noted two other twin moms using their feet, and again this made me nervous and depressed. It seemed so primal. I doubted my ability to soothe with my arms, and it looked like it might take all four limbs. Birthing the twins would signify not a respite, but rather a transfer of responsibility to my breasts and toes.

After the formal part of the meeting ended, everyone milled around to chat, and several women approached me at the snack table, where I was gobbling a poppy seed muffin, even the stale bottom.

One mom offered me a bag of maternity pajamas, just like that. Another said her nausea also trickled into the second trimester. A third woman came up to me while I brushed crumbs from my bump.

"Where's your other baby?" I asked her with a weak smile.

She wore one infant in a giant wrap contraption and gestured behind her at another. The sweet grandfather had the matching twin.

Then she spoke. "I hated my pregnancy, too. That's hard, if it's something you fought for. But you can hate your pregnancy and love your kids. It's not the same thing."

"Thank you," I murmured.

"It gets so much better after they're born. For this time, you have to hold them yourself. After, there are other arms."

I nodded, trying not to cry, though the tears that leaked out felt slightly like relief.

I had tried to say this to Ken, but even the closest person in the world to me couldn't understand as well as this stranger. She scribbled out her information on a slip of paper. She didn't know me from anyone, and I put the paper in my wallet, precious as currency.

I hadn't yet seen any immediate advantages to having twins. People talked about the "permanent playdate at age two," but that seemed remote, or the "awesomeness of having only one pregnancy," which made me mad. Now, in tucking away that woman's number, I recognized another gift, one I had overlooked, one I could enjoy without waiting: this pantheon of moms. They weren't amazing in the external "I still work out every day and I breastfeed *and* bring home the bacon and then host a party for ten" pregnant way. They were amazing in the deeper sense, the internal way, the way of people who *get it*. It was the opposite of competitive. We were all in a mess together, and there wasn't room to condescend, the borders between us less important than all our common ground.

At home, I looked at my calendar again, this time looking forward. I marked the next meeting, two weeks away.

WEEK TWENTY-ONE:

DOCTORS VERSUS GOD IN THE CASE OF MY TWINS

In the dark of morning, with a renewed sense of listlessness, I rose for the fetal echocardiogram in San Francisco. I groped for my glasses, ponytail holder, snack apple, and plastic bag, then followed Ken out the door without a glance in the mirror. My look was "effortless"—literally: black maternity yoga pants, with the panel shunted under the bump, and a black dress draped like a tent. I'd put this on at bedtime, seven in the evening, and crawled under the duvet. What was the difference between "clothes" and "pajamas," anyway?

It was surprisingly easy surrendering vanity, drifting to indifference. After a mere week of partial bed rest, I'd found the fashion equivalent of late-stage hypothermia, when the freezing makes you numb, dreamy, and you let go, snoozing into the snowbank. Especially for doctors' appointments, who cared what I wore? They met me without pants! To them I was a half-naked lady with a giant bump, a crucial if clunky accessory to gestation. I did not paint my toenails pink. I couldn't see them. I did not shave my calves. I couldn't reach that far down.

Sleeping in the next day's outfit saved me thirty minutes, since it took so long to change. The bump had grown to the point where I had to hold it as I moved up and down, while my knees creaked with pain and my fingers slipped. Waking up dressed added up to hours a week, time I could spend napping, or lying on my side. Dressing nicely (as in jeans) may have meant dignity and self-care, but for the echocardiogram I wanted polyester, in a dark shade that wouldn't show smears of clear jelly. I would be the hot dog, in a Zen way, and when they held that squeezable condiment bottle over my middle, I needed a comfortable bun. To this end I also kept two pillows in the car, one to shore up my bump and one to cushion my head, which I tilted to the window.

As the sun rose, we crept through traffic toward the Bay Bridge. Ken was at the wheel; I clutched my belly, moaned through potholes, and cursed at the mayor, the governor, the state of California, and the BMWs that cut us off. I stared out at the half-built, new bridge, which ran parallel to the actual one, and which would be earthquake safe, unlike the one we were crossing. The old bridge was too rigid and would crumble under stress, whereas the fresh one had a single anchor and complex flexibility. Those of us living in the Bay Area were waiting for that safe passage to be completed, just as we were waiting for the Big One. I felt this way myself, that my rigidity could not endure, but neither could I construct the better, stronger self I needed.

"Remind me again why?" I asked, referring to the echo-cardiogram.

"We like information," Ken said.

"Also the other thing," I added.

"Superstition." Even Ken had agreed we couldn't push our luck. What if we declined the echocardiogram and something happened? As with our decision to do the CVS, we worried we would always look back at our cavalier moment as the place where we could have made a difference. Regret avoidance felt protective, the way insuring your house made it seem less likely to burn, flood, fall down, or get robbed.

Dr. Abrams had been more blunt about the need for tests. "You don't want to ruin your life."

Less jarring input came from Dr. Silverman, who had told us if they did find a heart problem, we could line up surgeons to be present at birth. Fun as that sounded, we needed to rule it out, or so we hoped. Insurance likely wouldn't cover the procedure, but how could we make that calculation? Thus, another day, another doctor.

"IT'S LIKE AN ASSEMBLY LINE," I grumbled, as Ken dropped me off at UCSF's Building 400 for check-in. "Or the DMV."

"I'll meet you inside, okay?" He blew me a kiss and left to go park.

At the first desk, a guy examined my insurance card and waved me past to the next station. I imagined this system of gatekeepers helped eject the uninsured, shunting them into a separate, even slower labyrinth.

In the stage-two cube, a lady with wire glasses processed my information with surprising speed. "You're already in our system," she said.

I'd consulted their much-feted fertility doctor before Dr. Abrams, a woman who hadn't even looked me in the eye as she'd cheerfully rated my chances of conception at 1 percent. I wanted to pop by that office and boast, *It's twins*, but she was probably busy helping nicer, calmer people.

Stage three was lumbering to the restroom, which turned out to be too small for my pregnancy. To let me pass, two women on their way out flattened themselves in the narrow corridor, as if they themselves were twins getting born. In the stall, I almost couldn't rotate to get my butt on the toilet. Finally, I managed a ten-point turn.

In the lobby again I spotted Ken, legs crossed, *San Francisco Chronicle* folded. It took forever to traverse the floor, like wading through high water. The actual procedure would be in a separate wing of the hospital.

"They want me to take my pants off here, before crossing the street," I told him, in my best deadpan. "To save the doctor time."

"Ha," he said.

We moved at slug pace toward the sidewalk, me huffing, Ken breathless at the drag. Even in our dating days, he'd had to adjust to my gait in high heels—considerably slower than his rocket-burst steps in rubber-soled vegan shoes. I wasn't the only one who had to constantly wait; he was often waiting for me—waiting for me to finish up in the bathroom, waiting for me to mellow out, waiting for me to walk twenty feet. He was waiting for the birth of our children, and waiting for the return of his wife.

Through a maze of elevators and hallways, we found the pediatric unit. When we reached the floor, the air felt dense with emotion. It smelled like something I couldn't describe: the heartache of parents, the courage of sick kids. I stared straight ahead, terrified to look left or right into any semi-open rooms, as if they might vacuum us in, as if the spaces themselves hungered to be filled with suffering. Even as I tunneled my gaze, there were glimpses of posted crayon art, a child behind a curtain. I suddenly found I had a lower gear, and sped up for the first time in days. We beelined for the fluorescent-lit waiting area, a glassed-in cube crammed with toys and empty of people.

Ken took out his Purell and rubbed his hands, as if to absorb a prayer. Then we waited. I stared at my beloved iPad, Ken at his laptop.

"Why don't they have Internet?" I whispered. "I'm missing the *HuffPo*."

"Let's leave," Ken said, tapping away.

"I'll go get the car." I flopped back in my chair.

Thirty minutes later, a nurse told us they were finally setting up our room. "Someone borrowed the machine. We had to go find it on the top floor."

We smiled and thanked her, but inside I boiled. It sounded so inept and casual. I still wanted to believe that hospitals were highly organized hives of perfection, despite continuous evidence to the contrary. I pictured someone on the top floor having used "the machine" for some frivolous purpose, scanning someone's pet hamster.

Finally, a woman in hot-pink nurse pants and a matching hot-pink hand brace summoned us. "I'm Denise, your technician," she said, holding out her unbraced hand. She looked maybe twenty-nine, with straight brown hair and blue eyes. I liked her immediately, figured she wouldn't wear that nearly neon color if she were a harsh person.

The room was small and dark, Denise in fact friendly. "Hop up on the table. Let's have your belly."

"Keep my pants on?" I asked.

"Keep your pants on."

"Wow, this is a first."

There was a benefit to all this hugeness—you could practically see the babies through my stretched skin. I smiled, lying back, not even thinking how this was supposed to take an hour or more. Someone on the phone had said three hours, but I'd learned to ignore these estimates.

Denise slathered up my bump and got to work. I felt dizzy and asked for a pillow to prop me slightly sideways, so as not to crush the fainting vein. It felt awful, the gizmo on my skin, like being poked with a cooking implement, but I let Ken and Denise lure me into a grand distraction: our dogs.

Picturing Friso's prancing white form brought me halfway out of myself, out of my own repetitive thoughts. I couldn't imagine the babies yet, but I could perfectly conjure our puppy, with his snorty sigh, fluffy coat, and kibble breath. "He smells like a little farm," Ken liked to say, and we'd inhale his mild stink, like the crazy dog people I never thought we'd become.

Here's something I learned about twin pregnancy: it helps to hold pictures in your mind of what you truly love, focus through the static of fear on the cherished faces: your pup, your partner, your babies inside. With your mind's eye, you find your heart.

In the exam room, when Ken massaged my leg, I relaxed even more, trying to breathe deeply through the pained, tickling sensation of the scanner on stretched skin and smushed organs.

It lasted a little over an hour. By the end, I turned fully on my side, panting, proud I'd avoided a tantrum or meltdown. As with my slept-in outfit, the bar for my behavior kept getting lower.

"So, you really can't tell us anything?" I asked Denise, knowing she wasn't allowed.

"No, sorry, I like my job too much. But Dr. Grady will be here shortly, right after I go over this with her."

"Great." We thanked her. I studied her mouth for twitches of news. Nothing.

Then began the wait, again. Ten minutes, twenty. Thirty minutes, forty.

"I'm hungry," I whimpered.

Ken came back from the nurses' station with a jar of swizzled, tube-shaped cookies.

I crammed one through my frown.

Finally, Denise reappeared. "Dr. Grady is tied up with someone else, delivering devastating news. You might as well hit the cafeteria."

Of course she didn't reveal the devastating-news part, but I imagined it with complete certainty. This proved that such things happened. I felt my first real rush of fear about the echocardiogram. It was into the void of waiting that the reality of it rushed—there was no reason that we would be exempt from babies with heart defects. Cranky resistance and persistent denial were not bulwarks against fate. We'd rushed by those rooms to escape sickness, as if speed and motion would keep us safe. Just as we didn't dally on the Bay Bridge lest the earthquake hit, the stillness of a clinical wait made me feel like a target. At the ugly heart of impatience was terror. If I knew for sure the babies would be okay, who cared about the extra hour? I would stay all day.

All this fear uncorked my pent-up whining, along with hunger, and I whispered repeatedly to Ken, "I hate this place. I hate them." In the irrational state helplessness provoked, I thought the doctors themselves would decide our babies' fates, not just read the film. Of course, I'd feared doctors for years. In the murky layer of unconsciousness, they were actual gods, languid and capricious.

Ken squeezed my hand and left to get us food—a stale-looking roti for him, a pasta salad and a tub of tofu for me. I cranked upright on my seat, where now I really had spent almost three hours. "I want to know."

"Me, too," Ken said.

Then came Dr. Grady, who had stunning hair—long, blond, thousand-thread-count shine, striking even in my unhinged state. Was she having a hospital romance? She looked like someone who would marry a Kennedy. She definitely did not sleep in her clothes, *and* she had a medical degree on top of that. Her locks didn't even suggest excess effort; she just had great genes.

I longed for our babies to have good genes too, not for their hair, only for their health. The doctor took Denise's seat. *Be a bitch, be callous, but give us good news.* It wasn't about superstition anymore, or diplomacy. I wasn't numbly sliding to sleep but wide-awake and quaking, stuck halfway across this unstable bridge to even more shaky ground, motherhood.

"I'm so sorry," she said.

I stopped breathing.

"About being late!"

"No problem," I lied, as if I'd been waiting patiently, which was maybe why they called you a "patient"—wishfully, as a suggestion.

I'd surrendered my vanity, and now, amazingly, I felt another kind of giving up: my own sense of suffering burned down to something much more core. I didn't notice myself, only that I wanted our boys born howling and strong, and without a team of cardiac surgeons standing by with terrible tiny tools.

After another squirt and more scanning of my bump, Dr. Grady hung up the device and leaned back. "Everything's fine."

Fine. We would take fine! I didn't even fish for "good."

Ken and I gripped hands. "Oh, thank God," we said at once.

Lest we be too relieved, she explained that things could still go wrong. At this age, the babies had holes in their hearts, which didn't always close correctly. "As of today, though, it all looks normal."

"Normal," Ken said to me when she left.

"Normal." We high-fived, grasped hands.

We drove home in quiet.

"We could have skipped that," I couldn't help saying.

"We learned something important," he affirmed.

"Turns out waiting with pants is hard, too."

Week Twenty-Two:

Too Big To Fail

After checking the calendar to confirm that, yes, I'd reached only week twenty-two, I half-reclined on the living room sofa, slurping my breakfast shake of banana, kale, peanut butter, and powdered whey, before nibbling through two hard-boiled eggs. Ken was headed to work, and the day stretched in front of me like black ice. I could barely see it but sensed the hazards ahead. How would I get around? What if Friso needed help? He'd trotted off somewhere, probably to poop on the new rug in the rec room. Lately he'd had accidents, to my chagrin and guilt. Walking him had become difficult. My hips ached, my skin strained, the bump throbbed. My finger joints felt too loose to grasp anything, and if I dropped the leash, it hurt to bend or lean. I often left spoons on the kitchen floor until Ken got home.

I tried to focus on the beautiful word Dr. Grady had given us: "normal." I decided that day I would do normal things. I would work on the grant proposal I was contracted to complete, like a normal woman doing her job. Then I would drive to the Gourmet Ghetto, a few blocks away, and get fresh English muffins at the Cheese Board. So normal.

As I stepped from the car, squinting in the noon sun, a short-haired, be-sandaled woman immediately entered my airspace.

"Ooooh," she said, eyes pointed at my middle.

I lamented not having brought sunglasses so I could glare openly. Instead I stayed glassy, offered a faint smile.

"When are you due?" she asked.

"Not until December."

"Oh my," she said.

Five minutes later, someone else said, "Expecting?"

"No, I'm just obese."

Actually, I said yes.

"Soon?"

"December."

"Wow," she said. "I'd like to write you a check."

No, she did not say that. She shuddered.

Only one woman with a small boy nailed it and asked, "Are you having twins?"

"Yes," I said.

"Do they run in your family?"

"No."

"Were you surprised?"

"How about you? Did the condom break?"

No, I stayed polite.

"We were surprised," I said, no smile now.

As I plodded along Vine Street, I felt amazed by my size, my slowness, my sick stomach. I couldn't fully cross Shattuck on the "walk" cycle—as I plodded, sweating, the skinny white stick figure changed to the red flashing hand. Lost in the striped strip of street, traffic idling as I crept toward the far shore, I felt as if twin pregnancy were the dress rehearsal for extreme old age, a preparation for death.

Maybe that was the crux of hating the hugeness—the loss of power. Once spry, I now relied on the alertness and mercy of my Berkeley brethren not to mow me down in their cars once the light turned green. The vulnerability was excruciating. Some careless cyclist or skateboarder could crash into me. I'd be tipped sideways like a tanked cruise ship, faces looming over me while an ambulance wailed in the distance.

Only in the retrospect of my massiveness did I recognize the power that had come with a trim, fit body—the option of sexual power, in part, but more so the freedom of feeling my inner and outer selves matched. Now, even the phrase "inner self" seemed meaningless, like it had been cleared out for *actual* inner others, people I hadn't met yet but planned to serve forever—my two babies.

Most of all, I hadn't recognized until now the power of being nondescript. I'd always been able to move about invisibly, under the great cloak of the majority, which meant unthinking whiteness and easy health. Not only had I fit appearance-wise into a particular social group, I'd always been brown eyed and brunette in a way that made people think they'd met me before. If anyone called out to me on the street, it was "Susie!" or "Beth!" I used to joke I had a missing twin. Now, even at twenty-two weeks, I'd grown conspicuous. If I'd been trying to let go of the privacy of wearing pants with doctors, I'd now also lost the privacy of public space.

As I reached the corner, a guy waiting for the bus greeted me with a grin. "How about those Giants?"

"Great," I smiled back. "Feeling giant myself!"

In reality, he commented on my body in a robotic monotone. "Pregnant."

I pretended not to hear.

Near the corner, I approached a homeless guy on a crate, who chanted his usual request to passersby. "Spare some change. Spare some change. *Street Spirit*, right here. *Street Spirit* and a smile."

In the parallel world where I was earth mother to all, I always gave this guy dollar bills for his newspaper. In this world, where I was flawed and tight-fisted, I did not. This being North Berkeley, the panhandlers already got tons of attention. Gray-haired women in expensive clogs discussed Buddhism and offered prayers; bearded men with bicycles brought them lattes and goat cheese pizza.

The guy went on. "Spare some change, spare some change, anything at all, after you take care of your business."

The people in front of me blazed past him. As I reached this human tollbooth of conscience, I smirked self-consciously. So few people were like the woman in San Jose who had approached me in a restaurant, my dread mounting with her every slow-motion step, though she reached me and said only, "You look so beautiful, gorgeous," then smiled and left. It had made my night.

Now, perhaps this was my karma for treating homeless people as invisible: that I myself should become a spectacle.

It seemed endless, trying to pass the *Street Spirit* guy, like being stuck behind a plodding car, except I was that car. I wondered if I'd be obliged to speak an actual "no." As I reached the call zone of his crate, the man stopped shouting to gorge on the sight of me. I didn't look back, but I felt waves of both fascination and pity.

"Take it easy," he muttered.

He really said that. I nodded, surprised.

I smiled.

A minute later, I reached the ATM, where a line snaked almost to the neighboring flower shop. Three people in front of me exchanged head-jerky glances.

A woman spoke. "Do you want to go first?"

"Yes," I said.

They feel bad for me, I thought. *Even homeless people feel bad for me!*

This could have been a coincidence, but no, I passed another panhandler on the opposite side of the street, and he, too, interrupted his litany and muttered, "Congratulations."

The freak show of kindness didn't stop there. I had to get back to my car, and halfway across the interminable intersection at Vine, I noticed the boxy white cab of a parking ticketer, whom I liked to call parking demons, causing Ken to use his Darth Vader voice to read the vehicle name: "INTERCEPTOR!"

Now, I shouted to the demon from the distance. "Wait! Wait! I'm coming! Please wait."

This lady looked up, took me in.

"How far along?" she asked.

For a moment I thought she meant the meter, or how far

through the crosswalk. "Oh, this," I said, glancing down at the bump.

"Yeah, that. Some things you can't hide."

I looked down again. My feet were certainly hidden these days. I thought I was wearing flip-flops, but I couldn't say for sure.

"Three months left."

She looked surprised.

"Two boys, due Christmas."

This seemed to simplify it, and I could see her face slowly do the new math. She zipped off.

I got back in the car, poleaxed from twenty minutes of errands. It seemed hilarious that a few months earlier I'd been eager to wear maternity clothes, as if others—and perhaps I myself—needed convincing that I was pregnant. In Las Vegas I'd wanted to stand out, to show, while now all I wanted was to blend back in.

Week Twenty-Three:

Orgasmic Birth Is Not a Twin C-section

I t's the best-kept secret—orgasm during labor," Dr. Young said, though only in the parallel world. I had in actuality heard this many years earlier, from a woman on ABC News discussing a childbirth documentary. However, no one suggested this might happen with twins during my planned C-section.

"We'll schedule you for December," Dr. Young said in the hallway of their office after an exam—the usual ultrasound, plus an icky swab.

Dr. Abrams joined us. "Right in time for the tax break!"

Ken and I laughed like such a crass thing had never occurred to us, though we had already discussed this at length. Of course we wanted to keep the babies in the oven as long as possible, but a 2011 birth would save us thousands of dollars. Happily, our refund aligned with medical protocol of surgical delivery at thirty-eight weeks. We'd have some extra cash, if not an orgasm.

The next day, Dr. Young called with more exciting

news. We now had an exact C-section date: December 29, 2011, at ten o'clock in the morning. If we made it that far, both Dr. Young and Dr. Abrams would be present for the birth. "Otherwise, some random jackass from the hospital kitchen will do it," Dr. Young explained, though of course she said, "Another doctor from our practice will cover."

I didn't worry too much about a total stranger making a major incision in my abdomen, because I didn't have a choice. What's the point of feeling disempowered by something already a given? Okay, I felt disempowered by givens all the time, but not by the C-section.

I figured I'd already become "one of those moms," part of an alarming trend of women who preferred to control the timing of birth. I couldn't even claim a high-powered career. I liked knowing the babies' birthdays and counting the days until I could stand again. It seemed fine that an unnatural pregnancy should conclude on similar terms.

When I hung up the phone, I felt elated. The C-section wasn't only my plan, but the doctors', too. They really believed these two babies would come. In this reaction I recognized the skepticism I couldn't yet shake, and how out of touch I'd grown with the bigger picture. In living hour to hour, nap to nap, cupcake to cupcake, I'd lost sight of the ultimate end: having two boys. The fear was like a blindfold. Now I was allowed to peek.

I decided to go to the twin parents' group, and even took a dedicated shower, then changed my clothes. I could step out of my pregnancy bubble and listen to the moms. I could let myself consider the stuff that mattered *after* the birth. What did infants do all day, anyway? Maybe I could find out.

As I parked by Bananas, I briefly remembered my original horror at the Twins by the Bay crowd: the babies outnumbering the adults, and the crazy ways they got fed. Now it seemed strange that a woman using her foot to rock a car seat had freaked me out. I couldn't wait to use my feet! Even to see them would be a treat. This time, I walked into that room with many of the same women, and they looked brave, and cool, and composed. I didn't focus on breasts and double snaps. Instead I noticed one woman walking across the room, and another with a cup of coffee. *They can pop in and out of their chairs! They can drink caffeine!*

There were two other pregnant women—one the single lesbian mom, and one I'd never seen. The Angelina clone had had her babies and was back in her normal skinny jeans. Everyone else was in varying degrees of stretchy apparel, surrounded by the usual mass of blankets, pillows, car seats, and strollers, all of us camped for two hours of Twin Baby Woodstock.

The new pregnant attendee, thirty-seven weeks along, talked about the pending delivery. She wore cropped khaki pants and a floral top, and her bump seemed wider than a singleton's but not so crazily jutting as mine. "I don't know if I want the epidural. Something in my spine. Yikes."

"Do you have to have one?" the discussion leader asked.

"If they switch from natural to emergency C-section and there's no epidural, then they knock you all the way out."

I vaguely understood that "all the way out" wasn't ideal, but neither did it seem so great to be basically awake during the C-section. I worried the epidural wouldn't be enough. The doctors were all blasé about the surgery. Dr. Abrams called it "the zipper," and Dr. Young mentioned "a bikini incision," as if the first thing I'd do afterward was prance on the beach in a stringy two-piece.

The single-mom-to-be had reached the full and amazing thirty-eight weeks, and she, too, looked more normal than I did, in jeans, and also a laterally squashed-out bump. "In my case, they want to induce. I've heard forty weeks is better, though after thirty-eight weeks increases the odds of stillbirth."

The lawyer mom answered her from across the room. "Can you talk about this with one of your doctors?"

"The perinatologist gives me the creeps."

"How about your OB?"

"Dr. No-Name is supposed to be good, but he has no bedside manner." A few other women nodded—these doctors were all known. "He's the only one really open to natural birth for twins."

Though I'd been continuously exposed to its fans, I didn't see the big deal about natural birth. I knew the facts about faster bounce-back and fewer complications but didn't pursue them, since my own course was set.

My friend Tess joked that the glory of a C-section was "preserving the downtown." I felt already there was too much traffic there, what with the constant exams. I would avoid the mother of all jams in that area—two twin boys trying to get out. An aunt had mentioned that the babies' heads wouldn't get smushed and the surgery itself wasn't that bad. Of course, I knew it would be harder than the fibroid extraction, but I didn't expect our children to come out my belly button.

The negatives floated my way, too. "It's so industrial," one friend said. I'd heard others say things suggesting babies born by C-section, thereby missing labor, would be lazy their whole lives. I didn't believe that having a baby pounding through my parts would instill a work ethic.

At the twins group, no one spoke judgmentally about this kind of birth or that. Instead, one of the moms summed it up perfectly. "Ultimately, the doctors are going to insist on doing what's safest for everyone. This isn't an experiment for them."

Some babies—in fact, many—came early and were fine. One woman said she worked until thirty-six weeks and had an emergency C-section the day she stopped. Another mom's babies arrived three months early and spent nearly the rest of term in the NICU.

Yet another woman I hadn't met before came in late, trudging slowly, pushing the requisite double snap. With short, dark hair, she looked round and swollen beneath a draped shirt and wide pants. She chimed in on the topic. "I gave birth with no drugs whatsoever."

Everyone congratulated her, and she listed the details of labor and dilation and, of course, the long spell of waiting, waiting, waiting.

I wasn't sure whether she was boasting, until she talked about the experience of the Oakland hospital. "They didn't have a double monitor, so I couldn't walk around while in labor. So that was fun. And there wasn't a room for four, so we got stuck with another family, which was also a blast." It took a while to recognize the sarcasm in her upbeat delivery, and by the end of her story I felt happy for her, to have that note of pride in her voice. She'd earned it, not only by giving birth but by keeping her humor.

Even with all the mishaps, she'd claimed some power in the whole thing, which was more than I could say I'd managed in my pregnancy so far. It was inspiring.

I blurted out my news to the group, deciding to be honest. "I have a C-section scheduled, and I'm excited."

Here's what they didn't say to me, as others eventually would:

I'm so sorry.

The recovery is hard.

Breastfeeding is hard.

You'll bleed as much.

It's like being gutted.

What they did say was, "Congratulations."

It wasn't about painkillers or orgasms, work ethic or mashed heads. These women in the twins group knew how much I wanted to be finished.

I wasn't just "one of those moms." I was also one of *these* moms. An awesome thing to be.

WEEK TWENTY-FOUR:

DOCTORS WITHOUT DEGREES, HEAL US ONLINE

I n January 2010, when Sully Sullenberger landed his packed
plane on the Hudson River, I couldn't stop watching it on
YouTube. It looked like one of my worst fears, yet everyone
walked onto the wings, into waiting boats.

The same hopefulness now crept into my pregnancy, as I
found a website claiming babies born in week twenty-four
would have a 90 percent chance of survival, with medical
intervention. It would be a potential disaster, and a NICU
trauma, and the website itself was based in the UK, whereas
the American sites had a grimmer view of such small
preemies. But some part of me thrilled at the thought *viable
babies—even if only in England*. My job was to keep them in
the oven another ninety-seven days. I felt more excited than
I had at the initial news of pregnancy. In my fear-warped
view, this new kind of tenuousness was great progress. I
didn't dare expect a smooth taxi to the gate of parenthood,
but I could allow myself to believe in a water landing, and
tugboats nearby.

It was also the week their eyelids came unfused.

"Unlike a singleton baby, they will look at each other!" I said to Ken.

"I'm not sure about that," he mused.

"Because they're so close?"

"Not many photons in there."

I didn't care. No one could say open eyes weren't progress. My mood also soared in the realization that I hadn't chundered for almost a week. I moved the white plastic trash can back into Ken's office–man cave, where it could continue not to contain the room's Clif bar wrappers, plastic bags, and date pits.

The biggest problem was still lack of sleep. I tore myself from my TV binge and cuddle time with Ken at about 8:00 p.m., as I disintegrated into heartburn, dizziness, and thoughts of doom. Then I crawled into one of three spots— the daybed in the nursery, the queen-size bed in our bedroom, or the papasan chair against the wall. I switched between these stations all night, usually after a detour to the toilet, and dragging four or five pillows. With each transfer I slowly levered myself down, gripping the bed board or bamboo frame, then reassembled my padded moat: one leg over Longfellow, bump on cheese-shaped wedge. All this I bolstered with square foam pillows, one under my head, one over, one in front, and one in back. After two minutes, bottom hip crushed beneath the weight, I'd flip over in a slow arc, rolling over the fainting vein, then once again reinforce the whole nest. I felt like Sisyphus with cushions.

One night, midturn in bed, I fell onto my back, then couldn't move. Arms flapping, I finally reached the cell phone to call Ken in his room. "I'm stuck!"

"Coming."

A moment later, he rolled me back onto my left side, where I could sometimes feel good. I never forgot I was pregnant, though. Miracles can suck, I reminded myself. Those people on Sullenberger's plane probably didn't appreciate landing on a river during the descent. Did other twin moms sleep blissfully through the night? I hadn't heard of any of them, not even in England. Even when my body cooperated, there was still my mind: waiting for the birds to hit the blades.

ANOTHER DAY, an enormous box arrived on the doorstep, with my mother's return address. I sliced into it with an X-Acto. Inside were three Allergy Luxe pillows outfitted in Ralph Lauren covers, and two pairs of tiny socks attached to a piece of REI cardboard. A note on top read: *The pillows are for me. The socks are for Bernie and Bertie. Love, Moo*

I suppressed a twitchy feeling at her explanation. Maybe she thought I'd try to wear the socks myself, on my earlobes. I didn't know why the pillows bothered me—obviously, it was more than a few cubes of bedding. My mother was flying out to visit at the end of October. I'd begged her to come earlier, then made her promise that before she booked a flight, she would check the dates with me.

Instead she had simply e-mailed me an itinerary—a ticket confirmation—for a week she'd selected.

"You promised you would check in," I said.

"I called, but you didn't answer."

"I was out for *an hour*."

"The seats were filling up."

My face heated. "I hope Karen doesn't mind that you're going to be spending her birthday here," I said, trying to triangulate some of my agitation off onto my sister.

"No, I checked with her. Maybe we can all go out. Or maybe have a little party at your house—cake and presents?"

"I'm on partial bed rest, remember?"

Why was she so concerned about Karen? My sibling angst reared up, with its companion worry that my twins would always feel this, too. Not so deep down, that was what pestered me about the pillows. I wanted them for myself, and the silliness of this only made me feel worse. I knew the pillows were for my mother's own back woes, not a statement of indifference. Yet I wanted her, in the most literal way, to help cushion my pregnancy.

She, however, had moved on to the more interesting topic of the grandkids themselves, and her voice took on a whole new level of excitement. If my ongoing complaints about pregnancy didn't register, the fact of two new children certainly had. She thought I should be reading to the unborn twins. If their eyelids were unfused, they could also hear. "Try Dr. Seuss. Read to them every night—they'll hear the cadence."

On this topic she e-mailed and called continuously, repetitive as a Seuss character herself. "Have you gotten the Dr. Seuss book?"

"No book, Mom, but feel free to send us one."

"Oh, no, I don't have it. You'll have to send Ken to the library."

I'd told her many times I rarely visited the library— borrowing a book felt like rescuing a pet for only two weeks, and I hated waiting for books on hold. I had to have my stories forever.

Later she sent a clipped article, cleverly entitled "Double Trouble," about how two-year-old twin boys were "doubly monstrous." Penned by their grandmother, the article explained how she could no longer handle grandtwins' antics and had decided to stop babysitting. The author sounded proud of her decision, as if that was why her daughter had had two babies in the first place, to stick it to Grandma in her golden years. Was my mother telling me she wouldn't babysit? I didn't think so. She loved small kids and seemed more excited about grandchildren every passing week. I, on the other hand, felt slightly terrified of what twin toddlers might dole out. It had been hard, I'd found, to find positive stories about twins.

Perhaps I was a tad sensitive. If I were overly codependent, my antenna always cruising the signals of other people's emotions, my mother's tendency was to tune them out. My hunger for her undivided attention was part of the pregnancy, as much as the vitamins, the protein, and the bed rest. Would I have felt the same way with a singleton pregnancy? Surely my "mother issues" would have bubbled up as well, but the weight of twins meant I had fewer courses of evasion. I couldn't travel or exercise, those healthy modes of distraction. I couldn't hep myself up with coffee or calm myself down with wine. I couldn't even go out for dinner or stay upright for reality TV. I couldn't pretend that I wouldn't potentially face every single thing she had been through as a parent and a person. The vulnerability of having two kids—I understood it now, though I wished I didn't.

The real question was why our interactions continually startled me. My mother loved me. I even asked her periodically, "Do you love me?" To which she'd say, "Of course I do. That's a stupid question." She'd been generous with me over the years, but she wasn't one to fly flags of affection, sing songs of praise. Of herself she'd even said many times, "I don't do emotion." Twenty-four weeks into my twin pregnancy, I could barely do anything else.

My friend Linda came later that week, as she often did, with rice, chard, tofu, and peppers, which she sautéed in our kitchen while I sat on a stool, pawing at my bump, sitting on one of my mother's pillows and stating for the thousandth time how much my body hurt.

Linda listened to me over the wok's whispery hiss. She never issued dire warnings about never sleeping, never getting my body back, or never having fun. Now, she glanced up from the steaming vegetables and said, "It's going to be so worth it, though! I can't wait to hold your babies!"

The glee on her face shocked me into a moment of gratitude. Babies! Why did I keep forgetting that part?

Over dinner, which I devoured with near-tearful excitement, Linda and Ken chatted about quantum physics, about which she'd made a short documentary. She'd also worked on a film about IVF. Through the infertility, she'd been the only friend who seemed to *get it*.

I listened to my husband and my friend talk, trying to wrench myself into the present, but the present mostly contained fears about the future. When Ken got up to make tea, I told Linda what I'd read about preemies, and the images I'd seen online.

"If I'm this uncomfortable, I don't see how this can keep going."

"The misery doesn't mean that. You should have seen my sister, and that was only one baby."

"But the NICU. Those babies. Those wires."

"If that's what happens, you'll get through it. I don't know how it's all going to unfold, but I have faith in the goodness of the outcome. This time of not knowing will pass."

Her kindness soothed me more than any tangible gift. I had mothers and sisters all around, orbiting, if only I cared to unfuse my own eyes, allow the photons to let me see.

WEEK TWENTY-FIVE:

Waiting Without Pants

On a Monday morning at Dr. Silverman's, one part of my pregnant self looked fabulous: my cervix.

"It's long enough, right?" I asked Marcy, like a guy with size issues.

My pants were in a ball on a chair in the dim room. Over a wrinkled black tunic, I wore a nonmaternity, fleece zip-up jacket, hiked above the bump, which gave it a ridiculous cropped look. Bits of oatmeal shellacked the soft fabric, since a napkin could no longer span the hillside. I clutched a bed pillow I'd brought—mine, not one of my mother's—in hopes of stabilizing the bulge.

Marcy hung up the ultrasound wand, tossed her gloves, and nodded in agreement. "Your cervix is a whopping four point six centimeters."

She didn't say "whopping," but I felt pleased. Here was yet another pregnancy issue I'd never heard of before I'd conceived twins: that a shortening or "incompetent" cervix can signify early birth, so an alarming measurement might lead to bed rest and/or a tidy set of stitches called "cerclage." Despite the charming French-sounding label, I dreaded the thought of such sutures, so if the rest of me was huge, then at least this crucial piece of internal anatomy followed suit. My body had gone off the rails—the aching inside-out navel; the cracking, stained skin; the gurgling two-way esophagus —but the dolphin held the gate.

"That's awesome," Ken said, trying to cheer me up. We had two appointments that day, the thought of which left me miserable. Usually, one doctor's visit took a full day's recovery. I'd been dreading this twofer all week.

Next, Marcy wielded the second scanner over the jellied bump, which felt like a giant bruise. When she hit my belly button, the *f*-word escaped my mouth.

"Sorry," I said immediately.

"Don't worry—I hear that all the time."

"Really?"

"Yeah."

"From twin moms?"

"Everyone."

"It's not you. I'm a total dinosaur."

She laughed. "Now, *that* I haven't heard."

For once, I didn't turn my head to the screen. If I looked, I would see those little faces and be flooded with love. I didn't want to cry.

My mother was so right. I should be reading Dr. Seuss, not teaching them the word "fuck." They could recognize my voice, my scent. "Mother" would be the smell of Zantac and the swearing of a sailor.

Dr. Silverman came in. The babies were one pound,

eight ounces, and one pound, six ounces, which sounded so substantial. Mere weeks earlier, they had been a couple of ounces each, smaller than the amount of liquid TSA let on a plane, those teeny bottles you can barely squeeze. Now, they were a handful, as people loved to say of twins.

Our doctor went on—their heartbeats were good, growth good—yet his usual smile was missing.

"Your levels of amniotic fluid are high. Still in the normal range, but high."

"But normal?" The addition of "range" made me nervous.

He bobbed his head ear to shoulder. "It's something to watch."

"But it's fine?" I asked, hoping we could negotiate.

"Let's see next time."

Ken and I were silent when he left.

"That's their job, to sweat the small stuff," he reminded me.

"I thought that was my job."

"We work as a team." Ken handed me my balled-up clothes.

"I can barely get my damn underwear on. Everything beneath my bump is like the fourth fucking dimension."

"That's my girl."

BACK IN MY PANTS, I hung heavily on Ken and we cohobbled to the deli around the corner, a four-legged dragon from a Chinese New Year parade. Inside, I sank to a chair to study the chalked menu, then ordered scrambled eggs, a buttermilk blueberry pancake, and the ultimate indulgence: decaf coffee.

If I were to found a religion, the rituals would include this rich, brown, caffeinated drink, set on an altar, in a lidded steel mug. For nearly twenty years leading up to infertility, I'd woken before sunrise to finish a cup of coffee in silence. This elixir of wakefulness lifted me from fogged muteness to clear thought. After two cups, I could speak again, the Little Mermaid reclaiming her voice. With coffee, I could write.

For years I had scooped out the grounds the night before, inhaling the scent of the earth's chocolate, the little whisper of the tiny bits against metal a breath of faith; I intended to get up the next day, participate in life. I'd traveled toting my own coffee bags and water heater. At home, I stored packets of liquid espresso for the earthquake kit. I'd never planned to go without.

Now, it was supposedly okay to have a cup. It still scared me, but not as much as having two vaginal exams in one day without a treat. Having finished at Dr. Silverman's, we were headed to Dr. Young's.

"It's like a taste of the old country," I whispered, sipping the thin brown liquid.

"You are funny," Ken said.

"There is still some pleasure in this world," I said glumly.

With the divine bittersweetness on my tongue, I felt it all well up again, the sense of sacrifice, and the ambivalence at what we faced as parents. It would be years before I could sit in the morning and savor quiet, the exact flavor of coffee. Without caffeine, how would I handle the exhaustion of caring for newborn twins? How would I breastfeed them, anyway? I knew about football holds, and "breast friend" pillows, and the dreaded pumps, but it seemed over-whelming. How would I carry two babies to the car and strap them in their seats? Wouldn't that take an octopus? Where would we go, anyway? Most of all, if I felt so petty now, so nervous and unsure, how would I ever manage to mother my sons?

Suddenly, a buttery smell in the deli seized every synapse. I whipped around, like Friso at the slightest crinkle of a treat bag. An egg, cheese, and bacon sandwich, on a croissant, loomed within reach. It was vanishing into the mouth of a heavyset man in black leather biker attire, with multiple spike piercings in his face. He was clearly unaware that a massively pregnant woman was about to snatch breakfast from his fingers.

I managed to speak instead. "Excuse me. Can you tell me what that is?"

"It's the breakfast special," he said, in a squeaky voice for someone so tattooed. I felt as if we'd swapped identities. I sounded hoarse.

I lumbered back to the counter. "Can I change my order to the breakfast special?"

"Sure," the owner said, because he was nice, or because I was huge, or both.

The anticipation of this meal soothed my nerves and my apprehension at yet another exam, while my fears about actual parenting shot to new heights. My cervix was fine, but my priorities were not. How could I be ambivalent about two children but thrilled to the point of drooling about weak coffee and an egg sandwich?

"DO YOU HAVE A two-for-one on that circumcision, or is it per baby?" I asked.

The receptionist at Dr. Young's had handed me a contract for prenatal care, which included costs for the birth: $3,000 out of pocket, plus $350 for the C-section, with extra for circumcision, listed at $450.

She smiled. "The circumcision is per baby."

"Oy," I said, summing it up, and better than "fuck" for tender fetal ears.

Down the hall, I did the paper-cup pee routine. Then a nurse in the hallway led me to the scale. "Hop on," she said.

"With my jacket?" I asked, harkening back to the day when a pound-or-two difference mattered.

"Sure," she said.

The scale squeaked beneath my feet. The weights slammed to the right.

153.

153!

I was forty-seven pounds heavier than I'd been on our wedding day, with weeks and weeks to go. The only thing that would still fit was the veil. We should have registered for fertility treatments.

In the exam room with the cool oil paintings in boxy frames, I peeled off my stretchy pants. Almost right after, in came Dr. Young. My bare butt hit the paper, while a little sheet draped on my legs. Dr. Young, energetic as usual, opened my file for the new results from Dr. Silverman, which had beat Ken and me across town.

Then we were on to the exam, and I did my best to

scramble up my brain and leave my body behind. It still hurt —it was crowded in there.

Dr. Young sighed at the end. "We can't do the fibronectin test today because the lubricant from Dr. Silverman could give a false positive."

This test gave hints of preterm labor, and Dr. Young seemed disappointed. I was elated. One fewer procedure downstairs! At the same time, I knew every test was a safeguard, and the medical help an absolute privilege. This conflict only stoked my foreboding.

After two doctors' appointments, I felt wrecked, exhausted physically and emotionally. Having two babies would be like this day. I would take care of one child, then do it all again.

"Any concerns or symptoms?" Dr. Young asked.

"Hugeness," I said immediately, trying to sound saner than I felt.

I reserved the unbridled crazy for Ken, the "I'm doomed," "Is this a mistake?" or "What if I die?"

"What if I get an infection and they cut off my arms and legs?" I'd asked Ken in the middle of the night. I'd read about that last scenario in O, the Oprah Magazine. The woman had soldiered right on, concerned only with getting prosthetics so she could care for her children. My own fear about that outcome was far more selfish. I wanted my body back whole.

Dr. Young smiled. Though petite, she didn't look small. She managed to have a deep voice and calm manner while also being cheerful. "I was wondering when you were going to really pop," she said.

"Can I do this? I mean, will my frame carry twins?"

"Yes, yes."

"It's so horizontal," I said, glancing at the bump.

"You may have stretch marks."

Actually, she said, "You will probably have stretch marks," but I didn't like taking on this kind of prediction from doctors. No one knew! I planned to defy them!

"I'm worried because I had that fibroid surgery. They made an incision in my belly button. What if it bursts?"

"It won't burst," she said, sounding certain.

I tried to believe her.

"Though you will probably have an outie."

"Ugh," though I didn't think an outie would land me on *Oprah*.

"Any cramping, pain, discharge?" Dr. Young asked.

"No," I said faintly, realizing that some of my concerns were unsayable. *I'm not sure about having twins. I'm not sure about having kids at all, despite IVF. I'm not an earth mother, I'm not a strict mother, I might turn out a lazy, ambivalent mother, and it scares me to death.* My babies were now viable—but was I? These doctors were looking for something wrong in my body, but my problems were upstairs.

Week Twenty-Six:

Twins Plus Puppy

September felt like fall, a shift to crisp air, though Berkeley stayed sunny and bright, a rebuke to my sacked-out self. The seasons didn't change much on the sofa. Half a year had passed since the night I'd dreamt of two blimps plunging into an ocean and turning to submarines. It must have been an omen of twins, a notion that intrigued me and lit a little candle of excitement, that these twins were not only a product of IVF but also something spiritual, that they had *chosen* me, as I had chosen them.

Either that, or the blimp-submarines were a sign of how my front (and back) would balloon outward, then droop down.

The bump had expanded in all directions. On the north side, it pushed my ribs outward, fusing my breasts to the upper dome. At the southern slope it formed an outcropping that I called the Overhang. At first it was annoying. It made sitting more awkward and driving nearly impossible. Then the Overhang grew ominous, threatening to cover my hipbones and rendering nearly all pants obsolete.

When my father came to Berkeley for a weekend visit, I did my best not to cringe when he greeted me in the foyer with, "My God, someone blew you up with a bicycle pump!"

I knew he meant it playfully, and I quelled the urge to erupt. Besides, within a half hour, I'd guided him to a stepladder and spackle, babbling about household repair. Any lingering tension from the Tahoe visit got caulked up like the holes in the walls and topped with a fresh coat of white, jobs he took without pause or complaint. Maybe my father and stepmother didn't *get it* when it came to the pregnancy, but they didn't give up on me either, didn't hold a grudge. Or maybe the fact of twins had obliterated everything else, though it wasn't that they magically erased past conflicts. Rather, their pending arrival made it impossible to focus on anything but the future, and all that required of the moment at hand.

Neither did my father balk at finding the basement "guest room" a pile of maple planks, recently harvested from the sidewalk with a sign marked FREE BED FRAME. With a drill, screwdriver, and wrench, he built it through the afternoon, while I hovered nearby, useless. We chatted about his time in the army, decades ago, and the book about grammar he hoped to write, which he planned to call *Me and Her Went to the Mall*.

"Grandsons," he'd say, about once every hour. "I like the sound of that."

The second day, he installed blinds and hung pictures. The third day, he bolted together our bassinets, yet another project Ken and I had let languish.

Once, in our old house, we had taken months to replace a lightbulb in our kitchen, either wokking veggies in the dark or going out for $5 stir-fries at Oriental Express. It felt luxurious, somehow, to spare ourselves a two-minute task, and then humorous to see who would cave first and fix the light. The unfinished nursery was different, a symptom less of whimsical laziness and more of frightened exhaustion. We were waiting again, this time for certainty. In spite of my former feng shui rampages, getting too avid about the babies' room seemed like tempting fate. Tempting fate to do what, we never asked. We didn't want to know.

My father had none of these issues. Practical and hardworking, and despite the long career as a DC lawyer, he still saw himself as the small-town kid with a paper route, the first of his family to go to college. He had a Yankee practicality I could fake but knew I lacked. I loved this about my dad, how he did what needed to be done. When I griped about a jury summons, he'd say, "It's important to participate in this civic process." When I moaned about the hassle of changing the oil in my car, preparing tax returns, or even paying bills, he would say, "The cheerful acceptance of ordinary tasks, the slow accrual of completed deeds, adds up to a kind of love."

Actually, my father was too sensible to make poetry of a trait so ingrained, but he would say, "Oh, *Kathryn*. Just do it," in a tone of amused tolerance and steady conviction that always got my ass in gear. Here's something else I learned about twin pregnancy: when your double baby bump sprouts an Overhang, it's time to get your ass in gear. If you can't, be thankful to those who can.

Now, with two bassinets assembled, I could suddenly picture what they were meant to do, how those tiny, serious faces from the black-and-white ultrasound photos might someday gaze back at us from the mattresses. Two finished beds brought it home: twins.

With arms folded, my father must have seen it, too. "By golly," he declared.

"No shit," I said.

That's what we really said. The rest had been spoken with metal, paint, and wood, and with the labor and the finishing. When it came time for him leave at the end of three days, I didn't want him to go. We eddied a long time in the foyer. Friso tried to block the door, and my father, age seventy-one, got all the way down onto the hardwood to hug him goodbye.

THAT NIGHT, I cuddled Friso, nesting in the papasan, basking in the contentment of a successful parental visit, right up until my hand grasped a soft, cold patty. My eyelids shot open as my brain identified what my fingers held: dog dookie.

"Ken, Ken!" I shouted, as if the chair were in flames.

"What?" He leaped from bed, reaching me in seconds, plastic bag in hand.

If I was waiting without pants through this pregnancy, Ken was hurrying with bags—barf bags, grocery bags, even my girlie handbags, which were too heavy to carry now without tugging at my guts.

"Friso pooped in the chair!"

Ken threw on the lights, squinting at the brazen deposit. "I can't believe it."

"Me either." I heaped the sheets, lugged them downstairs. With Friso crated and sullen, I got in bed with Ken. That was it for sleep—nothing like grasping crap while dozing to leave me not only wide awake but churning with irrational thoughts. Dark waves crashed through the flimsy walls of my mind. *How can I walk the dog when my legs are like water sausages? What was I thinking getting a puppy? If I can't take care of him now, what happens when two babies come? How will I be a mom if I can't even take care of a dog?* We'd gotten Friso at the trough of infertility, when the waiting and the not-happening had seemed intolerable. Of anything we'd tried, only the puppy had brought solace. He'd made us parents, at least in my eyes. I wanted to care for him the way I would a child, and his lack of training seemed like one more hue on the vivid spectrum of my deficiency.

Around dawn, a practical thought appeared in the froth, and I clung to it against the undertow. I could take Friso to Metro Dog, the doggy day care that had helped us during IVF. That way, I could do what I most needed to do: stop worrying and rest. That plan lasted until Ken left for work and I found a circle of yellow vomit on the man-cave couch. On a hunch, I checked our bed and found our white floral sheets decorated with random poops and pools. I picked up Friso and drove to the vet.

Once there, I settled onto a bench, full of waiting-room déjà vu. *I don't have to take off my pants for this*, I thought, almost surprised. Instead, a half hour later, I watched Friso endure the thermometer in his south end while he whimpered, worse than going to the doctor myself. Friso couldn't rationalize about the greater good of having this done. At the same time, I realized that no matter how much I rationalized each medical procedure for the pregnancy, there was still an animal part of me that freaked out.

"It's some kind of massive infection," the vet said of Friso.

That evening, it took an hour for us to wrestle the prescribed pills into his jaw, Ken crouched with a bad back, me moaning with the Overhang.

"How many more nights of those pills do we have?" I asked, the two of us breathless on the kitchen floor, while Friso glared at us from the corner.

"I think you mean *years*," Ken said.

"The kids have to be easier," I said, doubtful.

"At least they'll shit in diapers!" he said.

"By the time they get to college, we will, too."

For three nights, Friso seemed okay. Day four he peed on the daybed and the rec room rug downstairs, then threw up on the deck.

Back at the vet, worn out and scared, I felt the same old flotsam and jetsam swishing through my head. *If we can't change a kitchen fixture, how will we change diapers for two years, for two babies? They're not lightbulbs—they can't just wait. If I hate taking one puppy to the vet, how will I get two babies to the doctor?*

After twenty minutes, the waterworks gushed and hiccups hit. I stared down at Friso's black eyes, his trusting expression, blocking out the surroundings, the hardness of linoleum, the people in uniform, the pulsing presence of those back rooms, with needles and prods and probes. I lifted him up, cradled him on my bump, glad for once of the extra-wide platform.

To my left, a man with a shepherd mix ignored me, but across the room, a woman with a black Lab shook her head. "This guy had cancer a few years ago," she said, ruffling the dog's head. "It was so hard."

I nodded, wiping my nose on my sleeve. I couldn't tell her that Friso had a probably-treatable infection, that I cried from fatigue, fear, and guilt, along with something else I couldn't yet name, a tingling feeling, a stretching not unlike that of my skin, but inside my chest.

"Being in that state doesn't make it easier," she added.

"Yeah," I croaked, forcing in a breath.

After the exam, the vet assured me they would keep Friso for the day and give him IV fluids, anti-nausea drugs, and a new antibiotic. Blurry-eyed, I got back in the car to head home. Instead, I veered off the freeway toward Oakland. I couldn't calm myself, but I knew where I might be heard. I could still make it to the Twins by the Bay group, an hour late, not that "late" meant anything in Twinland.

THERE SHOULD BE A SPECIAL label for a day when you cry in front of over thirty people, because once again, there I was, blubbering on the second floor of Bananas, with a roomful of moms, babies, and pregnant women.

Once seated, I came unraveled. "It's . . . hard." I couldn't say the rest: hard to stand, hard to walk, hard to sit, hard to eat, hard to talk, hard to breathe, hard to think, hard to believe it would turn out okay.

The badass lawyer mom was double breastfeeding again on all fours, and she listened intently, like she planned to win my case. Someone passed me a napkin, and the group leader asked, "What's been going on?"

I choked out, "My puppy is sick."

Not a single soul pointed out the non-baby-relatedness of this problem.

One woman, whom I knew to be recovering from the high forceps birth of her twins, nodded in sympathy. "We went through that with our dog, too."

"What did you do?" I sniffed.

"We got through."

"Our dog isn't even that ill," I confessed. "I'm afraid I can't do what needs to be done, even the most basic walk around the block."

"Where do you live?" one of the single moms asked. "We could come by and walk him."

"So could I," offered another mom, leaving me stunned.

This was so much more than just *getting it*. The busiest people in the world reached out to me, and to Friso, a dog they'd never met. Their kindness, their motherliness, went beyond babies. Here, the practical blended with the irrational into something beautiful. Maybe that was what the craziness and strain of multiples had given them, or what they'd found, or maybe created. Maybe I, too, would find an overflow of love, what I'd felt at the vet, that stretching in my chest, an expansion within. If you think having a dog will change you, try having a baby, and if that doesn't make you bigger in every single sense, try having two.

On the way back to get Friso, I made myself drive slowly.

At the vet, a woman in a white lab coat walked him out, his eyes droopy, his gait slow. With his chin in the air, he pressed himself against my cankles.

I levered myself down at odd angles to scoop him up, like my dad had folded his sore joints down a few days before. I stared into his puppy gaze, and I knew something I hadn't that morning. This wasn't like the fetal echocardiogram, where it had to be okay. There were no guarantees, for Friso, for me, for the babies. But I could harness the crazy, use it as fuel. Maybe we couldn't go around the block, but we'd go to hell and back if we had to. I knew, for the first time, I could be a mom.

WEEK TWENTY-SEVEN:

DOUBLE BABY SHOWER KARMA

At the news of a bridal or baby shower, my mother liked to say, "Blech. I hate those things. Just send a gift." If my father flew the flag of duty, my mother thumbed her nose at convention. For a few years after my parents' divorce, we'd often had an empty refrigerator, but we still had box seats at the Kennedy Center. It wasn't that groceries were beyond reach—to the contrary. Rather, beauty became the prime necessity, the core nurturance, in a time of despair. I understood this priority, all the more so as twin pregnancy demanded I focus on the purely practical, the dully physical.

My mother stuck to what moved her and labored to ignore the rest. A patron of the arts, she wore jeans to the donor galas, and as a tech tomboy, she practically prayed facing an Apple store. Once, in her brand-new red Prius, she tried to outrun a policeman at Dulles Airport. He was a bully, she said. She'd fled on principle, peeling out as he reached for his ticketing pad. She'd even taken her case to court—unsuccessfully.

As an adult I took pleasure in her eccentricity, which I saw as a joyful rebellion against the status quo. During my single years, she'd proudly told her friends of my sister and me, "My daughters are skipping their starter marriages," holding our choices in the highest regard. She never once made me feel like I should buck up or settle down, and after a breakup, she'd offer affirmation, counsel. "Don't marry anyone who hasn't been married before. You don't want to be anyone's first wife." My mother celebrated independence, and the maternal defiance that had buoyed me through hard times became trickier during smooth ones—for instance, while planning a wedding. It had seemed to make her shudder, and she'd declared her relief to live far away. An hour before I walked down the aisle with Ken, she was lying on her back in the grass, in her sparkling pink floor-length St. John gown, complaining that her stomach hurt. Her sister, my aunt Joy, in a tie-dyed turquoise jumpsuit, sat nearby, holding her hand. My mother and father saw each other about once a decade, and no matter how much Ken and I juggled seating charts, an event like a wedding caused colossal stress—for everyone.

Like my mother, I had also always disliked the ceremony of showers, especially the way they divided women into this camp or that, married or unmarried, moms or childfree. At baby showers, the Vagina Ladies exhorted the moms-to-be about latching and pumping, while the bored nonmoms milled and clotted in the kitchen. During the long unwrapping of blankies and bouncies and binkies, I'd made all the requisite noises of awe while privately mourning the end of an era. The days of spontaneous dinners were gone forever.

The new mom would only ever appear at the edges of a nap, through which she'd be checking text messages, or she'd bring the baby, and our talk would be lost to *goos* and *gahs*. It made me melancholy, the shower like a long goodbye.

Then, during the years of infertility, that wistful feeling shifted to something sadder, a cramping in my chest. I couldn't force the smiles or cheerfully answer the people asking if I had/wanted kids. Though I'd always questioned my mother's avoidance of this social obligation, I suddenly stopped going to showers altogether. In some cases, I took it a step further and even skipped the gift.

Now, I was about to have my own baby shower—for twins.

It made me nervous, the karmic debts unpaid.

My sweet mother-in-law, Sandy, had offered to host. Despite my undeservingness, thirty people RSVP'd yes. I kept checking the Evite, touched by replies. Many of the guests were Sandy's friends and Ken's family—but my friends were coming, too, including the childless ones, who surely grieved my freedom, as I had done to others before. A few had said as much. Those childfree-by-choice friends had been skeptical of my efforts to conceive and had greeted the news of twins with flat congratulations that might as well have been anagrams for "nice knowing you." With two babies, I couldn't pretend that friendships wouldn't change.

I wanted to post something crazy to the Evite, like, *Hey, you don't really have to come. But please do.* Pregnancy had stripped my solitude of pleasure. Once, my quiet time alone had felt restorative. Now, I counted hours until my next round of human contact. Anyone who wanted to celebrate, I wanted in our home, and I pined for the type of gathering I'd so recently shunned. It wasn't even the idea of a party that mattered, but more what it meant: that people would show up, even with doubts, not for a long goodbye, but for a long hello, to the babies on the way.

Sandy had agreed to have the party at our house in Berkeley, to spare me the drive to San Francisco and the possible vomiting, which had mostly stopped, but not completely. Ken and I cleaned the house for days, I at a shuffling pace, and Ken excavating his office—years of old receipts, New Yorkers, spit containers from DNA testing kits. Linda made two trips to Sandy's in San Francisco in her "free" time—once to help plan the vegetarian menu, and again to roll silverware into blue napkins tied with white ribbon.

Meanwhile, I tried to coax my sister to come to Berkeley the day before the shower, but Karen insisted she couldn't. "I'm spending that night with Mr. Temporary," she said, using a different but equivalent nickname, and a tone to suggest the date was immutable.

For all other guests, I felt grateful, yet toward my sister, I felt annoyed, as if she more than anyone *should* come and help. In my new understanding, I thought some friends would bail, but a sister had to stay onboard, like the crew of a sinking ship. Karen didn't love showers any more than our mother, and we'd often called each other after this kind of event to marvel about how long it took some women to unwrap gifts. First trimester, I'd been careful and nervous about her feelings. Now, I wanted her there, wanted her invested, wanted her in line, the way my aunt had helped my mother through the trial of my wedding.

On the eve of the shower, I ranted to Ken, "These boys share up to half of Karen's DNA. Two children with half her genes each basically equal one child that's fully hers."

"It doesn't work that way," he said.

"How does it work?"

"Your sister's doing what she needs to do, and you are thankful for that."

"Yeah, right." Sometimes these nudges toward lucidity from Ken worked. I went to bed wired, but not overwrought, and slept twelve hours.

I woke feeling vestiges of my former self, person-ish, rather than a faulty bread machine into which someone had mistakenly crammed two loaves. I slowly got dressed in the bedroom, pulling out my last fresh maxi dress, black and soft, billed as the Angelina, perhaps after a celebrity twin mom, as if by name alone the glamour could be passed to the short and stout. Over my shoulders I put on a white cotton cardigan with long front flaps, bright and clean, if a little Hare Krishna in its draping. I blew-dry my hair, the first time since IVF, and slathered on lipstick, a dark brown shade. I felt as attractive as my size allowed.

I looked at the clock: ten minutes to ten. Karen would be there soon, but the wait felt long, like nothing would be real until she arrived. Then the doorbell rang. Once inside, she went straight to work, the party pro: setting up chairs, arranging paper cups, putting out plates. Finally, she found me on the sofa.

"You definitely didn't sleep in that," she said of my dress.

"I didn't."

"You look good, Koofy." She smoothed the back of my hair.

I mushed my head to her hand, Friso-like. I knew she didn't have to be there at all, not for karma and not for blood, and that was what had made me so mad, the power she had to make or break my day. "Thanks for coming," I whispered.

Linda came at eleven o'clock with black bean–polenta casseroles and two kinds of quiche, spinach-mushroom and broccoli-cheddar. Ken worked all morning slicing melon and strawberries, picking up coffee from Peet's, setting out butter, hummus, and cream cheese.

Meanwhile, I lounged sideways on the couch. "I'm trying not to look like Jabba the Hutt," I told my sister.

"You are much more Queen Bee."

"Ha. I like that."

Then Sandy showed up with cakes, sandwiches, champagne, juice, and an entourage of upbeat seventy-something women. More people came in dribs and drabs, cousins and aunts and friends. Linda toiled in the kitchen, the Goldbergs clustered in the living room, and the writers gathered by the buffet. Tess wrangled Friso, who danced at her calves, flinging himself onto his back for a belly rub. Lisa drove all the way from Santa Cruz, Michelle from San Jose, Mija from San Francisco, on a broken foot. Everyone bore boxes, which my sister stacked by the fireplace.

I tucked into the broccoli-cheddar quiche, having a small orgasm in my mouth. I devoured three pieces, crumbs tumbling on my black dress. To anyone who asked, I talked about the topic that consumed me—managing the hugeness, what I could and couldn't do. When I pondered this alone, I felt martyred. In the company of others, I could almost grasp it was temporary, a side effect of twin pregnancy.

At some point, my sister corralled everyone. "We'll be opening gifts, but it will absolutely not go past two o'clock. At that time, there will be cake and champagne."

I wondered if people were as reassured by the time limit as we were. They drifted into the chairs, arrayed in a big circle in the living room. One by one, Karen carried in large boxes from Amazon, bright striped packages from Giggle, and endless bags with tissue billowing out and stuffed toys dangling down.

She handed me each gift, let me read the card, extract the item, and say once, "Ooooh, aaah."

"Okay, that's enough." Then she'd snatch it from my hands.

Our eyes met, and we laughed.

Just like there was no one else who would give me the double middle finger before sunrise, no one else could make me laugh with years of wordless understanding. If my twin boys could have this, it would all be worth it.

Ken snapped photographs but mostly hid with the men. People gave us swings, bouncers, wraps, rattles, clothes, books, toys, socks, blankets, swaddles, onesies, and more. My mother sent a double stroller, my aunt two car seats.

Karen gave us a travel crib. Sandy had bought us a glider, the one from Kid Dynamo where I'd soothed myself months before, after bursting into tears as I spoke of having twins. Now, like the chair itself, twins seemed a tremendous gift.

Then Karen led us to cake and toasts. Ken and I offered our gratitude, the only thing bigger than my bump. A picture of us that I would love was taken, perhaps the only image of me pregnant that didn't make me cringe. It was one of those moments where I tried to pause, to say to myself, *Notice this*. It wasn't about filling boxes on a calendar, or unwrapping boxes of gifts, or even checking off boxes of milestones. The boxes that counted were the rooms of home and heart.

People stayed. Linda loaded dishes into the washer. Karen took Friso for a walk. Sandy's friends lingered, finishing up the coffee. I tilted myself on my side, bump beneath a pillow, happily evading questions about breastfeeding.

Though Karen wasn't the last to leave our house, it felt over once she'd gone. Right before, she'd spent a few minutes breaking down cardboard, bagging the wrapping, squaring up the stroller.

"Did I do a good job?" she asked.

"Hell yeah," I said. "Mom would be proud."

We laughed and laughed, and not long after, our house felt full of stuff, though empty of people. Not for long, I reminded myself. Not for long.

Week Twenty-Eight:

The Twin-Parent Tribe

In the far corner of lightless level P6 of the hospital garage, I swung open the car door to scoot, slide, and grunt from behind the wheel. Once on my feet, unsteady in my clogs, I made a shocking discovery: I couldn't turn in the corridor between parked cars. I tried not to panic.

I'd come all the way to San Francisco for a glucose tolerance test to detect possible gestational diabetes, another malady to which twin moms are overly prone.

Even without a diagnosed problem with blood sugar, I felt myself about to pass out, wedged upright between two SUVs. I could barely comprehend this latest demonstration of monstrosity. Finally I walked out backward, stunned by the absurdity of it, glad for the privacy of the subterranean gloom.

Mercifully, the elevator lifted me directly to the lobby, twenty feet from the lab area. Even to my cranky, critical eye, it seemed like someone smart had planned this out. Then, at the first desk, the woman directed me to get my "glucose beverage" first. "Your hour will be ticking while you sign in," she explained. After that jittery hour, a nurse would draw blood.

"Shortening my wait?" I said. "I love you."

No, I didn't say that, but I did give her a genuine smile, the first of the day.

At a separate window, a youngish guy with a combed-up wave of hair handed me a plastic bottle filled with orange liquid. Its size and shape conjured a grenade. "Drink this within five minutes."

"Is it disgusting?" I asked.

"It's a little like Gatorade," he said, with a note of doubt, which he covered with further instruction. "If you leave the area, be back in fifty minutes."

"It would take that long to get in my car," I said.

"You've got what we call 'parade float pregnancy.'"

No, he didn't. He gave me a nod, unfazed.

I unscrewed the lid and chugged the bottle in under one minute.

"It's more like DayQuil," I informed him.

"I've never tried it," he said, admitting the obvious.

"It's not so bad."

As I plodded off, I felt both pleased with my imbibing and also queasy, as the mother of all head rushes slanted my vision. Why didn't they give us a slice of German chocolate cake, or a fresh-baked custard-stuffed éclair? They could command us to finish a box of Godiva in two minutes. I'd probably have to give all that up if I failed this test, so this should be a last hurrah.

At the next sign-in station, a burly man behind the

computer offered me water. "I have twins myself," he said, confirming my name and address while he tapped at the keys. "Grown up now."

"Really?" I instantly liked him—my people, like all twin parents.

"We'll get you in and out as fast as we can," he said.

I sighed in relief, woozy now from orange drink.

Here in the hospital, my hugeness incurred kindness and haste in the staff, and the usual staring from everyone else. The twin dad directed me back to the waiting chairs, filled with magazine-reading middle-aged folk, a video game–playing teenager, and a bevy of cane-grasping elderly whose collective mood seemed best represented by the diminuitive gray-haired woman who repeatedly asked in a plaintive tone, "Where's Dr. Wong? Where's Dr. Wong?"

I felt her impatience, her urgency, and looked around for Dr. Wong myself. After about five minutes, I felt like I might faint. I'd gone beyond coconut-icing haze into full-out dizziness. I waddled back to the twin dad. "Is there anywhere I might lie down?" In my previous life, I would never have dared such a request, but my boundaries seemed to be expanding along with my belly.

"Let me check. Can't promise, but let's see."

I followed him behind the counter, into a warren of curtained-off cubes, down the line of them. At the end, one stood empty. "Here you go."

Another nurse materialized to help me lower the reclining chair—a black leather beast with test tube–holder slots on each armrest. She didn't ask why I needed it, and gestured for me to settle in. It was like being led into the first-class cabin of an airplane out of cramped coach. I must have said thank you more than five times.

Alone in my stall, I flipped awkwardly onto my side to semidoze, using my pink backpack, and then my iPad, to prop up the bump, thinking how well it worked for that unintended use. A tech had closed the curtain over my feet, my toes beyond the hem.

Less than a year ago, I'd come to this same hospital to meet the surgeon for my fibroid operation. Outside the main entrance, we'd passed a sign that said LEAVE YOUR BABY HERE, with a picture of a bundled infant, as if it were simply a category of disposal, like paper, bottles, compost, trash. From the standpoint of infertility, I couldn't fathom the desperation of those women, as perhaps so many couldn't have fathomed mine. The hospital, the entire medical realm, seemed filled with extremes, and I viewed that "baby drop-off" as if through a curved and smashed mirror, distorted and alarming, and I'd wanted to knuckle-smack the brick wall at the unfairness of it all.

The second time here, the day of the surgery, I'd tried to keep my underwear on until the last moment. Despite instructions to remove all clothing, I'd worn it beneath the gargantuan paper gown they'd given me for the three-hour wait. I'd been hungry after fasting, and scared of dying, and had shed sloppy tears as I confessed to a nurse I wanted a cupcake. When my surgeons arrived to escort me down the hall, I'd had to swerve into a bathroom and chuck my contraband lingerie in the trash, even though it was a favorite piece, with lace and bows and trim. Still, that petty gesture had helped me feel in control, like I didn't really belong in a hospital, and that while I was letting people I barely knew cut me open, I had power over my own knickers.

Now, in less than a year, I'd be back here for a C-section. Assuming, of course, there wasn't a catastrophic earthquake the day before, causing all the bridges to fall, forcing a neighborhood dentist to perform the surgery and stitch me up with floss. I worried about scenarios like that more than I did about gestational diabetes, even though my mother had had it and one in three twin pregnancies wound up that way. Plus, I hadn't exactly shunned sugar. In addition to the assigned vegetables and proteins and grains, there had been pounds of chocolate almonds down the hatch, bars of Scharffen Berger dunked in peanut butter, chocolate-ginger cookies from the Juice Bar Collective.

Drifting in and out of sleep in that chair, I noticed a rare sensation—the absence of panic. Once, this scene would have horrified me: the cubes, the strangers, the needles, the vials, the glimpses of infirmity. Now, worn out and run down, I felt linked in sympathy to everyone else. I hoped that woman in the waiting room had found Dr. Wong. Like the twin dad, she was my people, too.

I listened to snippets of nearby conversation, between techs drawing blood and those having it drawn. One guy was a student at the University of California, Santa Cruz . . . another guy grew up in the Mission . . . a young voice, a sonorous voice, was a phlebotomist in his third month . . . I enjoyed my private eavesdropping cell, wishing I had this much privacy everywhere I went.

Finally, about five minutes until my hour expired, a

woman with radiant latte-colored skin and pale pink reading glasses appeared and introduced herself as Amora. She whipped together the blood-drawing paraphernalia, and I barely watched, noting only out of the corner of my eye that my arm was being tied up with one of those off-white rubbery strips, then stabbed with a "butterfly needle," which they should have called a "bee sting." My blood was barely mine; I shared it with the boys, and the doctors, and whoever asked—happy hour at my elbow.

Somewhere in the course of the extraction, Amora told me she, too, had twins, now twenty-five years old.

"Wow, you, too," I said.

"You have boys or girls?" she asked.

"Two boys."

"They'll be best friends! My son says he feels naked when he's not with his brother."

I soaked up her words, an excellent trade for a vial of blood.

AFTER THE HOSPITAL, elated if light-headed, I drove four blocks to Mom's the Word and parked in front. I wanted a reward. I quickly slithered from the grasp of an unfamiliar salesgirl into the skilled hands of Sarah, the woman I'd met the time before. Even in the third trimester, my unbridled consumerism showered my system with endorphins.

Sarah recognized me through the bulk. "You are still tiny. It's all baby! *Babies*, I should say."

"It's mainly the middle, right?"

"Totally."

She brought clothes to my cubicle, while out from the next dressing room came another woman, who looked only slightly pregnant—a different species, as if she would be giving birth to an acorn.

Nevertheless, we exchanged electric good wishes, acknowledging the stages we were in. I thought how different this was than the first, competitive round of shopping months ago.

Sarah brought pants that didn't fit—boyfriend jeans, black cords, yoga leggings. The Overhang rode low, so "pregnancy panels" sagged on my hips, verging on plumber's butt or worse. Sarah didn't give up. She simply whisked away the rejects, which I slobbed onto the floor, unable to lean down.

Then she appeared with a final pair of pants. Not just pants, but jeans: J Brand, dark blue, with four pockets and "skinny" legs.

"There's no way," I said.

"Try them. They're a favorite with moms of multiples."

"Really?"

"They say they're the best."

After a few minutes, I got them on my legs, secured on my hips, and buttoned below the Overhang. In the mirror, I had legs. Those legs were in pants. Those pants were denim. Even tipsier than I'd been with the glucose, I not only bought the jeans but threw in a poncho-type sweater, vaguely aware that all my Target-loving, money-saving resolve had flown out the window.

"You have no idea what these mean to me," I told her. "The psychological boost."

The price tag shocked, and as I thwapped down my credit card, I pushed away the guilt. The second trimester would soon end—this wide, wide middle of the twin pregnancy, just like the wide, wide middle of my body. Clad in the jeans of my people, I had Sarah cut the tags and wore them out of the store.

Week Twenty-Nine:

You Must Be Due Any Day

"Got pants?" I said to Ken, over and over, through the hour-long drive to San Francisco.

"You do," he said, happy, I knew, to hear me upbeat.

"Let's park right in front. I'm feeling lucky."

"As you wish," he said, in his best *Princess Bride* voice.

We did park in front, high-fiving and picking through our quarters. Those San Francisco meters would make the time go fast, at twenty-five cents for ten minutes.

Inside, I lumbered to the bathroom to pee in the paper cup. I could now barely reach it under the Overhang, but I didn't care that day. I had pants. I walked as if the stares were those of admiration. Jeans! I'd modeled them for Ken that morning, singing, "I'm too sexy for my pants," swinging my arms forward and back, unable to move anything else.

"Your butt looks good," Ken had said, which felt like the most romantic thing I had ever heard, better even than the day Dr. Marion had praised my uterus.

"I know," I whispered, and by that I meant, no maxi

dress or muumuu. No pajamas on the town. No Vincent Gigante robe. I was a normal gal, having two babies.

The pants itched below the bump, but I didn't care. They stretched enough that I didn't have to do and undo the zipper, a crucial bit of NASA engineering.

Before leaving the bathroom, I drew two smiley faces on my sample cup to represent the twins, then lumbered out to the scale, where Ken and the nurse waited.

"He wants to see how much you weigh," she told me.

"I do, too. I think I'm starting to show."

She looked confused, then realized the joke. I must have been unrecognizable with a sense of humor.

"You think so?" She smiled.

"You can kind of see the bump." I turned to the side.

Placing her hand on the behemoth, she spoke gently. "You're showing."

After she took my blood pressure, Ken craned me up to the scale: 157.5.

Ken and I exchanged more high fives.

The nurse led us to the very back room, and Ken lectured her about the unsecured oxygen tanks in the corridor. "In an earthquake, those can become like bombs."

I felt a pang of pride that my husband was so smart about these things. Those tanks didn't even register in my visual field. Also, I enjoyed his efforts to enlighten the indifferent.

"Huh," the nurse said to him, and then to me, "Undress from the waist down, and Dr. Young will be with you in a moment." She handed me the cocktail napkin/loincloth.

When she left, I huffed, "I'm going to sit here for a few

minutes with my pants on. My time with this denim has been too short."

Ken looked at me kindly, accustomed to this outburst with every single appointment. He took a second chair.

After a few minutes, I shimmied out of my jeans. "There, I got some extra seconds."

My bare butt felt cold on the paper of the exam chair and crushed by the weight of fifty extra pounds, all the while on full display, facing the door.

"Do you want me to get you another of those covers?" Ken asked.

"Can you?"

"I saw a stack by those oxygen tanks."

A moment later, I eclipsed the full moon with the extra napkin. Then I heaved my feet crossways over the foot stirrups, trying to find a "comfortable position." I glanced up at the clock, dreaming of a Next Doctor app, where you could watch them wend toward you on your iPhone.

After a few minutes, Dr. Young breezed in, with a big smile and her usual aura of enthusiasm. I loved this about her, the lack of anything haggard or impatient. "How are you doing?" She sounded concerned, perhaps also baffled to see my mouth in an unfamiliar configuration—smiling.

"Feeling pretty good," I said.

She opened my chart. "What changed?"

"I got jeans."

She giggled. I'd made her laugh! This thrilled me, even if I seemed shallow. In addition to actually liking Dr. Young, more generally, I had shifted my sullen distrust of doctors to active people pleasing. I strove to charm and disarm. That way, they'd work harder to keep me alive on the operating table. I'd be that much more human as they screamed for the defibrillator.

I tried to sound thoughtful. "Seriously, some days I feel okay. Others, the world is ending."

She nodded, and I imagined she, too, was happy to see me in a better state. I seized the moment to be my actual, difficult self. "I have a question, though. I want to know why that swab test is necessary. I mean, isn't it kind of redundant with all the fancy pictures and measurements from Dr. Silverman?"

Dr. Young spoke with great patience. "These are different tests. With the fibronectin, if your test comes out negative, there's a ninety-five percent chance that you won't be going into labor in the next two weeks."

"Oh," I said. Had I been told this before? It sounded vaguely familiar. I'd been thinking of this test as a useless ritual. Her explanation made it seem kind of reasonable, even a good thing. Two weeks was lot of time to buy away from worry.

"That's information I like to have," she concluded.

I suddenly felt okay doing the test. "Can you tell me how long the swab will take, so I can count? I'm into counting these days."

"Ten seconds. That's after the speculum goes in."

"Ken, will you count backward for me?"

"Me?"

"Yeah, you, math guy."

So he held my hand, and I looked at his face, while he started. "Ten . . . nine . . ."

"That's too slow!" Dr. Young teased him, as he was lingering on each digit. "I'm better than that." It ended at four.

"That was so much easier," I said, still always evaluating, but not fighting.

"You *are* feeling much better," my doctor affirmed.

Then there was the regular cervical exam, involving hand and glove, which I minded much less, and there I was, back at the lessons of IVF, always negotiating the degree of discomfort, if not the fact.

"Any concerns?"

I braved a glance at the bump, the skin stretched to the limit, and my belly button a red slash on the veiny curve. "Is this going to pop?"

"No."

"It feels like it. I scratch all night, and the skin is so thin."

"That's not going to happen."

The Berkeley crate-sitting panhandler who'd once wished me well had now taken to saying, "Wooo-hooo, you about to *pop*!" So had the Bank of America security guard by the ATM, and a woman with a wretched terrier in the Holistic Hound. I found these exchanges jarring and now had to check with Dr. Young.

I reminded her of my history. "There was that fibroid surgery. Now my middle is like a sock that's been darned, and it won't hold. Especially my belly button."

"It will hold," she said, sounding sure.

I finally confessed. "Everyone on the street says to me, 'You're about to pop!'"

"Tell them to fuck off," she suggested.

No, she did not. But she did say, "It's amazing what the body can do."

We scheduled two more visits on the way out.

On the way home, I still grappled with my fear of rupture. No matter what Dr. Young said, I feared the babies would come early, a statistically relevant concern. That twins came early half the time, often with all the complications of prematurity, was a threat that lingered around the clock. The people not rude enough to say I was popping liked to say, "Due any day!" They broadcast my own terrors, the ones I hoped to escape, even for an hour, by going out at all. It was like walking down the street after a breakup and having people yell, "No one will ever love you!"

I wondered if I should stay home. One thing was for sure: these days, I felt more comfortable at the doctor's than walking around.

Week Thirty:

Twin Pregnancy is Titanic, Mother is Ice

Because twin pregnancy left me immobilized, I had time for conversations with my mother, both the real ones we had by phone, Berkeley to Bethesda, and the imaginary ones in my head, while I waited for sleep. In every case, I fumbled for the words that would allow her to see me, to grasp my experience, to make her *get it*. This had become an obsession.

"Twin pregnancy is different, Mother!" This I said on an actual call, a week before her scheduled trip to California.

"That could be true," she said back, lightly, as if I were a zealot, not to be encouraged with too much response.

"It is," I insisted and, when I couldn't get agreement, kept saying to her in my mind, right up to the moment her boots clunked up our stairs and the doorbell rang. I chugged toward her, the *Titanic* mowing toward ice. "I'm coming!"

Meanwhile, my mother frantically clicked the locked doorknob.

I swung the door open, breathless. "Didn't you hear me? I can't move quickly."

"I thought you said, 'Come in.'"

I exhaled, clutching the bump. "Well—come in."

She heaved a pod-shaped backpack over the threshold. We did not hug. It wasn't our style, and besides, I was too huge. "I was going to call you from the cell phone but decided I'd surprise you."

"I figured it was you," I said, while she fiddled with her bag. "I would help you with that, but, you know." I gestured once again at the bulge.

"Ken is at work, I take it?"

"Yes. Got your pillows in there?"

She nodded. She'd packed two more. My mother stood before me, looking ever youthful with short black hair, crisp blue jeans, and rubber-soled mountain wear on her feet.

I waited for her to say something about my pregnancy. *Look at you!* Or, *You are so big.* Nothing came. Even my father's "Wow, someone blew you up with a bicycle pump" seemed better than no comment at all. I wore the same dress I'd worn to the DMV the day before to pick up a handicapped placard, the floor-length gown that accentuated my pendulous midsection. While I couldn't tolerate strangers shouting and meddling, the much-craved indifference coming from my own mother felt like the very first stages of a chest cold. Even at the DMV, that hub of monosyllabic curtness, they'd been strangely nice, rushing through my application.

With all this churning, I said, "Can you please take off those hiking boots?" I knew she found our shoeless policy both taxing and dumb, but I was in no mood for extra sweeping, and if I could get my shoes off, so could she.

"I have to wear them inside, for my back," she said.

Pursing my lips, I directed her downstairs, listening to her suitcase slam against the hardwood stairs—*bump, bump, bump*.

"I'm supposed to avoid stairs," I said, to no response. I followed her down.

I wanted to show off the basement, how we'd developed the rec room. Perhaps I could impress her with decor, if not my girth. When she did not reject or show signs of trauma at the sight of her room, I rationed myself a moment's controlled pleasure, like a single organic walnut in a bag of nut dust.

I didn't mention that I'd sidewalk-salvaged the bed, nor that my father had built it. She might have praised the parsimony, but mention of my dad would have left only taint. Upstairs again, I loosed Friso from his crate, and he raced up to my mother, nuzzling her leg.

She leaned to pet him. "Aren't you cute!" She seemed to genuinely enjoy his white, fluffy head. "Aren't you soft!"

I chalked a victory, this one solid. My mother had been calling Friso "the dog," as in, "Please don't let the dog on my pillows." Maybe he would rally us through this visit, my twelve-pound pup.

In two hours, Ken would be home. If my mother didn't always delight in my admittedly dour company, she held my funny scientist husband in the highest regard. We both relaxed in his presence. While we awaited his arrival, we did not discuss my pregnancy, or the fact of pending twins. Instead, we gushed about our Mac products—my iPhone, for which I'd stood in line at the Apple store, and her old laptop, which she'd saved for playing Super Munchers. Then we mourned Steve Jobs, no less powerful a figure for having passed a week before.

"I can't believe he's gone."

"It almost doesn't feel real."

"Ken's been wearing jeans and a black shirt for days." Actually, he'd been wearing it for years, but now it was an homage to our family's prophet from Cupertino. "He's even got the beard."

When Ken got home, we decided to order Chinese takeout. My mother stared at the paper menu, fists clenched. This happened when the entrees exceeded $7 or seemed "fancy." An excellent cook, she didn't see the point of ordering out. It was often a matter of personal creed, an ethic drawn to extreme, the way she sometimes walked a bill to its destination, just to save a stamp. My great-grandma Betty, I'd been told, had done this in her jewels and furs. It had skipped a generation. I'd come to view takeout as sacred.

I tried to preempt. "If the prices disturb you, it's our treat."

"No, it's not that. I don't see anything."

"What would Steve order?" I tried to keep it light.

She stared at the menu, bereft. "There's no lo mein."

"There are other noodles—homemade at this place," Ken offered.

"Will you call and ask about lo mein? Otherwise, I'll get chicken fried rice."

With my father, I wanted him to take care of me. With my mother, I wanted her to be happy with what I could offer. I wanted her approval, whether it was for Chinese takeout or for two grandchildren from one stressful pregnancy.

After she finished her fried rice an hour later, I stupidly asked how her meal was.

"Awful. Bad. Boring." She sounded so angry, as if chicken fried rice had been advertised as the celebrated special. "There were barely any vegetables."

"Do you want some of our stuff—the moo shu vegetable, or eggplant?"

Vigorously, she shook her head.

I tried one more time to steer toward my twins. "I'm glad I can eat Chinese again, after that awful morning sickness."

At last, her face softened. "Karen used to throw up, too."

My pregnancy didn't come up overtly until almost bedtime. Ken had slipped into his office, and I shuffled to the kitchen to fill up the two water bottles I guzzled at night. My mother was at the dining room table with her laptop, and I commented how much my back hurt. "It's crazy, the constant ache."

"Can't the doctors give you some medicine for that?" She kept typing.

I slowly turned. "The only cure is childbirth. I had one doctor tell me, and I quote, 'Twin pregnancy is torture. Get used to it.'"

Never mind that Dr. Meanie's comment had enraged me at the time. Now I wanted her as my ally and authority. I had to show my mother I was deserving of empathy, even love.

"Torture," I said again, to be clear. "The doctor said."

"Hmmph," she said, swallowing.

I said a terse good night. In the bathroom, I brushed my clenched teeth with the electric toothbrush, which sounded like a buzzing bee between my ears. Before noon the next day, I could no longer hold back, as my mother went on about how she'd gained only seven pounds while pregnant with me. "I wore regular pants until the end, unbuttoning the top button."

I finally asked her, "Are you surprised how big I am?"

Without missing a beat, between spoonfuls of granola, she vented her truth. "You're not really that big."

"I've gained fifty pounds, mostly in the middle."

"What size were you before?"

"Like, clothing size?"

"Yep."

"I was a size zero."

"Does that even exist?"

"It certainly does."

"I thought you were more like a six."

I almost laughed, but crankiness trumped. "Mother, this isn't about dress size. I'm not fat—I'm carrying two babies— and you have no sympathy."

There, I'd said it. Like the rules of barfing, I had to accept it would all come up.

"I don't know what you're talking about." Her eyes narrowed.

"Like last night, you were like, 'Can't the doctors give you some medication?'"

"I never said that!"

"You did!"

"I didn't, and I never would." Her voice brimmed with outrage, sandpaper at the biggest grain, to erase me, or so it felt.

"You did." In most families, over time, everyone remembered things differently. In my family—both sides—shared facts lasted less than a day.

"What I meant was, haven't they given you any exercises?"

"Like, physical exercise? I walk. This isn't like a singleton pregnancy, where you can roll around and do yoga."

"That's not what Andrea and Anya said." There it was, coming up on her end, too. These were her two physical therapists, the ones who exhorted her to extra pillows and shoes indoors.

"Oh, is that what they said?" I shot back.

"They said there are exercises that can help you."

"How kind of them! I presume they're flying out to help?"

"I don't want to fight with you. Let's drop it." Her face looked hard, closed. It was out: I was to blame for my condition, the "torture" of twin pregnancy.

"So I guess your exercises have cured you of all ills."

"It helps."

I went nuclear on pettiness. "But you still have to wear boots in the house?"

"I don't want to talk about it. I don't want to fight. Case closed."

"I'm going to nap," I said, though I could barely blink, much less close my eyes.

IN THE NURSERY, I perched on the single bed, too churned up to lie down. I cued up my '80s mix on the iPod, randomly hit a song by Asia. To their anthem of electric guitars and pained betrayal, I crammed a Halloween stash of Reese's

Peanut Butter Cups into my mouth. I glared out the window, fully a teenager again.

Eventually, incredibly, I fell into a nap, orange candy wrappers crushed beneath me. I woke up to a stream of negative thoughts: *I can't bear it, I can't bear it.* I ranted to an invisible audience that included Ken, doctors, friends, and all those anonymous blogger moms who jabbered about miracles and breastfeeding. I mentally Skyped Dr. Meanie. *Yeah, you were right. It's torture.*

Staring at the empty bassinets, I calculated that I'd had no fewer than seventy vaginal exams in one year. I hadn't yet added up how many doctors this included—but, as a start, a random OB in Berkeley, the "1 percent chance" endocrinologist at UCSF, Dr. Brill (for the surgery), Dr. Abrams (also for surgery), six or seven techs at the fertility clinic, six or seven techs at Dr. Silverman's, and then Dr. Young, and also her colleague Dr. Torres. This calculation thickened the cloud of my morose mood.

I felt plastered to the bed, which made me think of my own mother at my age, the almost-forty mark. It was right when my parents had divorced—unwanted on her end, to say the least. She crawled beneath the comforter, and the ordinary pattern of days as I'd known it ground to a halt. The air was thick with sadness, murky as a churning wave, and I swam through it with her, suspended, her grief and mine merged. When my father came to pick me up every other Saturday, or halfway through Christmas Day, my mother burst into tears. I felt numb with guilt, leaving her behind. I still loved my dad, through the pained bafflement at his sudden absence. He seemed to regard their eighteen years of marriage as wrapped up by whatever they had signed, as if "the check" they were always discussing were but a restaurant bill. They were the pioneers of the 1970s divorce rush, carving out the roughest country, terrain that later waves of breakup immigrants learned to avoid.

Now, after having vowed to myself I would always be an on-the-ball mom, I was lying in bed weeping, barely functioning, fully irrational. For a moment, it all seemed linked —some old pool of grief to which I'd returned to drink, swallowing a belief that radical change meant not transformation but decimation. This insight didn't make me feel better but did crash me back to sleep, so my deepest mind could teethe.

After sleep, the anger dissipated into remembrance. This was an old tussle, the way it was with my mother and me. Threads of adolescence still pulled my adult strings. I felt bound up in her feelings. If my belly button was the physical scar, our link cut when I entered the world, there was also an invisible scar that existed from a later time. Still, my mother and I kept trying to make real contact. There was no version of history in which the *Titanic* and the iceberg change plans, give up, choose a safer course.

If I perceived her not *getting it* as a kind of harshness, I also felt that harshness whether my mother was in the room, or in the state, or elsewhere altogether. I suddenly understand why the kindness I received from others, as well as the comments I despised, shook me so hard. Half the time I was in dialogue with a phantom version of my mother, as a phantom version of myself.

Having her in the house, no matter the endlessly circling

conflicts, gave me a feeling of clarity, of separation. I couldn't spare a drop of energy for this ancient tug-of-war. I was forty and pregnant. At times, this blessing unleashed elements of torment. It was like the CVS, something to accept. I wasn't going to argue anymore.

BY EVENING, my mother had shifted to a quieter mode, too. "Do you want me to take Friso around the block?" she asked.

I nodded. "I would love that."

The next morning, she announced a plan to make lentil soup.

"That would be great," I said, worn out.

She even got herself to Andronico's on foot, came home with a bonanza of groceries. She wouldn't be subjected to the indignity of chicken fried rice again. We'd have a home-cooked, vegetarian, nutritious meal—the likes of which we hadn't seen since my belly got too big to stand at the stove or sit at a table. For half the day, she sliced vegetables in the kitchen. "I'm going to make some to freeze, too," she said.

As she tied an apron around her waist, I launched my 4:00 p.m. bed rest, and while Ken fetched measuring cups, spices, and pots, some bygone mother-daughter dynamic was restored—or maybe reinvented.

I realized I'd never rested with her there in the house. When she flew out to visit, I did my version of rolling out the red carpet and then insisted she walk it exactly as I desired. Once, I'd taken her to a play at the Berkeley Rep, then bristled when she'd declared that "the set looked cheap." Another time, after I'd hauled her to San Francisco to tour her through a museum, she had somehow slipped from my company, lost for an hour. I'd panicked, sprinting around to find her, as if I'd lost a child. As a helicopter daughter, I'd failed miserably.

Now, rather than "babysit" my mother, I let her tend herself.

The next day, instead of hovering, I headed out for the twin-parents meeting. Maybe my mother didn't *get it* about twin pregnancy, but I'd found a group of people who did.

Meanwhile, my mother made plans with Ken's parents, Joe and Sandy. This was another first—usually Ken and I chaperoned these get-togethers. They all agreed to go to Fatapple's for pumpkin pancakes.

The twins group was uneventful, besides the excitement of activating my handicapped placard to park right by the door of Bananas. Most of my pregnant compatriots had crossed over.

One of the single moms had two teeny babies in the standard stretch-limo double snap, and Angelina spread her little ones on a blanket. There was one other pregnant woman, who at thirty-three weeks was much smaller than I was. I envied both her progress and her reasonable size and tucked into an almond croissant.

A friendly mom came over with her new twins.

"You're at thirty, right?"

"Yeah," I said, glum.

"You have two more weeks until thirty-two, which is a big milestone, and then three more until thirty-five, and then it's countdown."

"But I'm realizing it's not going to get less uncomfortable, only more."

"The discomfort changes, though. It's always different."
I clung to those words.

FOR THE NEXT TWO DAYS, I continued to rest, and my mother kept cooking, filling the house with smells of sliced garlic, warm pasta, homemade tomato sauce. Our last night, she served plates of fresh spinach lasagna in the nursery. Ken and my mother pulled in chairs, while I ate in bed.

"Breech and Transverse are at it again," I told Ken, moaning with the hurt of foot and fist jabs but also excited by the sensation.

In a calm state, I knew they weren't seeds or grapes or yams or even flippered fish, but babies now, skinny and squirmy. I didn't have room inside me to nourish two infants and a grudge, so I let everything hard about the visit melt away. If the blessing of my pregnancy brought torment, the torment also brought the blessing of release. I hungered for my mother, and I let myself be fed. I savored every bite of the lasagna, the three of us talking about *Mad Money*, which Ken and I called *The Shouting Hour*, my mother a Jim Cramer devotee.

At eight, they went to go watch, while I hunkered in bed. Breech kicked low in my pelvis, hitting organs, while Transverse pummeled the top hemisphere, against my ribs. I rubbed the bump and, for the first time ever, felt them respond directly to my touch. That's what children and parents do: we kick each other from the inside. We define ourselves as separate and yet forever seek the primal bond. Finally, I yanked my shirt up. An entire forearm, elbow, and hand surfaced beneath my skin. I gasped, amazed by the intensity of it. Then the arm was gone.

I hobbled to the man cave. "I felt and saw *an arm* inside me." I sank to the couch between my mother and Ken, then bared the bruised bump. We all stared.

"I don't see it," my mother said.

"Wait."

We stared some more.

"Can I?" my mother said, hand over my middle.

"Sure," I said.

Down came her palm, gently, on the ancient scar of my navel.

Up came the arm.

My mother didn't move. She, who didn't "do emotion," looked like she might cry, with her mouth open and eyes distant. Then her face softened into awe, even joy. It hurt a little, her touch, but I didn't care. Just like the twin mom had said: the discomfort wouldn't go away, but it would surely change.

It's possible not to know what you are waiting for until it arrives, as it did in that moment in the messy man cave with Cramer clamoring from the TV. My mother's touch on the torn skin of my belly. Her trembling expression. A flashed glimpse of our future, as clearly as I saw my babies' beating hearts on each ultrasound screen. Loving these twins would steer my mother and me forward, a radar signal to guide through the rough waters and heavy fog. There was beauty ahead. The *Titanic* sank long ago. The iceberg melted. All that remained was so much treasure, waiting to be pulled to the light of day.

WEEK THIRTY-ONE:

TWO BABIES, TWO FLOODS

"Dr. Silverman will be in with results," Natasha, that day's ultrasound tech, informed us as she left the room, as if we might forget to wait.

"That wasn't bad," I told Ken.

"She gives good transducer," he teased.

"Totally."

We'd been giddy all morning, having left two black bean polenta casseroles on the car roof in the rush to San Francisco. When we'd parked, the pair of compostable takeout containers hadn't budged, despite headwinds, turns, starts, and stops.

"If our lunches can stick for the whole ride," I said, "so can our twins."

"I thought you were giving up omens," he said.

"I am," I lied. "Except good ones."

Swept up in the silliness, I'd forgotten to decode Natasha's face during the exam, through which she'd barely spoken. Nor did I notice that Dr. Silverman joined us without his usual brisk boredom. Instead, he wandered in and peered down at me. Still on my side, I craned my head over my shoulder to greet him.

"It's getting to the really hard part, isn't it?" he said.

"Yeah," I agreed.

"You can stay there while I do this." He readied the scanner and the bump.

I rambled. "At my twins group, I look at the other pregnant ladies and I think, *Do you even have a second baby in there, or are you here for the free doughnuts?*"

"Actually, it's not your imagination," Dr. Silverman said, hanging up the gizmo and rolling back his stool. "You've got an excess of amniotic fluid. You *are* bigger. And probably more uncomfortable."

"You have to tell that to my mother!" I fumbled for my iPhone.

No, I did not.

I asked in a squeaky voice, "More than last time, out of the normal range?"

"For Baby B, yes."

Discouragement rippled through me. "What does that mean?"

"We're going to monitor you more closely. Twice-weekly non-stress tests, and, depending on how that goes, maybe more."

I did not say, "Ugh."

He continued. "We don't have cause here. It can come with gestational diabetes, but you passed your glucose test. It also occurs with structural abnormalities, but we don't see any of that, and he's swallowing fine." Our doctor seemed reluctant but then added, "About half the time, we just don't know."

"In those cases, it's okay?"

"The main risk is that if your uterus gets too large, there can be preterm labor."

"Let me get this straight—you can have this and still have a good outcome?"

"Yes. Most of the time."

It wasn't enough to stanch the worry, but it wasn't nothing, either.

When he left, self-pity filled the vacuum left by his expertise. Why did I have to be larger? It was already two babies, and one of them had to have an extralarge sac? When that tide receded, in crashed fear. Here it was: the Complication. We'd been searching for it nonstop, this thing we hoped not to find. It was like the international hunt for loose nukes. Paranoia and optimism became indistinguishable, fused into one insane quest: find the danger first, save the world from ruin.

BACK AT HOME, I Google-binged. The condition of excess fluid, called polyhydramnios, came with trisomy and Down syndrome—stuff we had (supposedly) ruled out with CVS. It often led to early birth, just as Dr. Silverman had said.

I relaxed only with the arrival of Lori Colombo, massage therapist for moms and pregnant women, and the opposite of the Internet: physical, soothing, full of useful insights. On my side, on her padded table, I inhaled the chamomile oil, soaked up her strong hands, exhaled the endless tension.

"I just need not to think about the extra water," I told her.

"I'm sure it will be fine," she said.

I drifted toward bliss, until about halfway through the massage, when I heard Ken curse loudly. He called through the door, "A water main broke in front of our house. There's nothing you can do. Stay there." He wouldn't trouble me about the rapids gushing toward our yard, driveway, house, I'd later learn.

"Okay," I said, relieved.

Lori kept rubbing my back while, unbeknownst to me, Ken and two neighbors rushed fifty-pound sandbags into a makeshift levy to protect our driveway. Soon enough, sirens wailed, boots thumped, men shouted. I heard Ken, again, and lifted my cheek from the flannel sheet.

"This doesn't sound good," I said.

"Nope," Lori agreed, but neither of us disengaged.

A policeman-sounding voice boomed from the front of the house. "Is that your car? It might collapse into the pavement."

"Should I move it?" Ken asked.

"I will if you give me the keys," the officer said. "EBMUD is here now." The water utility had arrived.

"Should I be worrying?" I asked Lori.

"Nah," she said.

"Kathryn, do we have more sandbags?" Ken asked from the hall.

"Only the ones there," I said, giving up on rest. "Should I come out?"

"No."

A truck roared in the street as the massage finished. I wobbled to the front window, beyond which two men, our neighbors Tom and Lauren, hunched over the sidewalk dam of sand sacks. I'd been telling Ken for days, this bump was like having a fifty-pound sandbag strapped to my front. I clutched it now, my waterlogged babies.

The utility people stayed until 1:00 a.m., with floodlights and backhoe, while white spray erupted from the pit out front. In my bathrobe, I lurched out to stare at the muck and flood and mud. Neighbors had gathered, some with flashlights, some with wine, until everyone shooed me back inside.

I commanded myself not to think about water, or water breaking. Surely this wasn't as compelling an omen as polenta on a car's moving roof.

TWO DAYS LATER, I returned to Dr. Silverman's for my first "non-stress test." Tired, worried, and unwieldy, and to be on the safe side of the burst-pipe omen, I'd been googling "babies born at thirty-one weeks." As I clicked through pages, my fear of early birth faded, like a screen on low battery. Babies born now usually came out fine. In some dim corner of my mind, part of me wished ours might show up before the official time, just as Ken had on our first date all those years ago. He'd come early just to be safe, he'd said. *The babies are viable. They'd just be small.*

Then up popped pictures that killed my fantasy. One preemie looked like E.T., baseball head in an incubator, twig arms with clenched fists. His face pinched with strain.

Another preemie, mouth open as if in a silent scream, was covered in tubes and tape, curled, pink, and wrinkly beneath the glass. Even in my third-trimester insanity, I could see this wasn't worth it, not that I or anyone had much control. I had to soldier on.

For that first non-stress test, we entered a room with about eight cots, each cordoned off by curtain walls and flashing machinery. Our tech, Susan, directed me to "bed one," explaining it was better for those of us pregnant with twins.

"More padding?" I asked, still searching for the chance to relax.

"Rails," she explained. "So you don't fall."

"Shall I expose the behemoth?" I offered, when she'd latched me in. There was a seat belt, too—can't have the pregnant crashing to the floor.

"Anytime," she said.

The goop had been warmed, which I appreciated. An over-the-bump ultrasound marked the babies' positions: Baby A was transverse along the Overhang, while Baby B's head showed up on top. The rest of him wouldn't present.

"I feel him kick every day," I said, nervous that his body had vanished.

"Why don't you check over here?" Ken suggested, after about fifteen minutes of fruitless scanning, pointing to the top left quadrant of my bump.

Baby B's body appeared.

Then came the sensors, which reminded me of shuffle-board pucks, strapped on with white elastic belts, three in total, one for each baby, and one for contractions.

"Can you actually have contractions and not know it?" I wondered aloud.

"Absolutely. There's a lot going on. Sometimes women think it's just kicking."

"Hmm." I knew a kick—I could practically see it through my skin. The numbers spun all over the monitor. I moaned.

Susan reassured me. "That's good. Oxygen-deprived babies stay still."

At first the test showed willy-nilly data, one more useless medical hoop, I thought, when I could be at home, playing Temple Run on my iPhone or staring at the hole in the pavement left by the pipe.

"We'll do a bio-profile instead," she said, getting out the ultrasound again. "See, Baby A pumps his chest up and down. That's 'practice breathing,' a very good sign."

"What about the extra water?"

"There is some extra water," she said, but nothing more. She left us alone for a while, and the babies eventually calmed, giving a baseline, then squirmed, giving a measurement. Susan tallied their scores: Baby A got 10 out of 10, and B got 8 out of 10.

I felt a little defensive of B, as if I could lobby for extra points, but anything over 6 was good. I wiped the goo off the Overhang, careful of my precious jeans, which I hadn't yet washed, for fear of shrinkage.

"You have no contractions," Susan said, studying a curled piece of paper that looked like a fax. She then unhooked the many straps. "You are free to move about the cabin."

No, she didn't say that, but she did say, "How's your cervix?"

Full Vagina Lady now, I loved this question as much as I hated people on the street asking when I was due. "Great," I said with pride. "Holding down the fort."

"You're good at this," she said, and I rode the compliment all the way home, where I grabbed the TV remote control for some taped *Survivor*. I didn't think about water at all, even as the contestants got rained out of their shelter— not until a strange hissing came suddenly from our kitchen.

"That doesn't sound good, does it?" Ken said.

"Not really," I admitted.

Ken left. "*Oh, shit*. Kathryn. It's flooding. It's flooding!"

He raced ahead of me. I found him a moment later, hunched under the sink, ankle deep in steaming water, yelling. As water poured into the dining room and down the stairs, the fire alarm blared.

I left to get neighbors. By the time I reached the door, they had come to us, Lauren from next door, and Jen from two houses down. "We thought we'd better check on you guys," they said.

Ken ran up from the basement, the water shut off now but inch-deep on the floor. He and Lauren talked about pipes, made calls, gathered mops and towels. All I could do was watch. Our contractor, Carlos, showed up in a half hour, opening cabinets to find the latest busted pipe, this one ours, not the city's. EBMUD wouldn't come for this. A few minutes of flood damage would take days to repair, but at least we'd been at home. As with the pregnancy, we could only be thankful—whatever happened, it could always have been so much worse. In the new calculus, a small disaster counted as a blessing.

Lauren and Jen then hunted for their shoes, which Friso had taken hostage behind the sofa. After a while Lauren left, and returned with fans, while Carlos cut out drywall. He sliced through the basement ceiling while water and debris crumbled out in foul heaps. Not at all like an emergency C-section, I told myself. Not like polenta.

Through the scrim of fatigue, I felt awe that people kept showing up. I'd always believed that to draw the world in, you should be thin, look polished, have a perfect house and a winning disposition. Yet there we were, inundated with need, not to mention water, and not much to give in return but gratitude.

This, too, was an omen of things to come.

That night I piled pajamas, slippers, and onesies on the floor. It was time to pack a hospital bag.

Close to midnight, Ken relit the pilot.

Week Thirty-Two:

Like a Full-Term Pregnancy, with Six Weeks Left

Once upon a time, I thought getting pregnant meant scaling the mountain. Now, it meant being the mountain, except it didn't feel so Zen. You can't meditate if your underwear hurts, if it's simultaneously tight, saggy, and attacking your skin. Even the jail-striped maternity knickers I'd bought online drooped on my hips, while the elastic unraveled after one wash. The tiny rubber tentacles of the frayed "waistband" tickled and itched. It both caused and expressed feelings of frustration in this last lap of pregnancy, the slog of exhaustion, the pining for relief.

For months I'd been smug about my lack of stretch marks, slathering the bump nightly with overpriced cream from a pink-and-white tube. Now, lumpy red streaks had erupted in bands across my belly, especially around the center, and also down low, around the ever-burgeoning Overhang. It was as if someone had plowed it for farming, then abandoned it to drought. Touching it scared me, between its limb lumps on the surface and the unblinking monocle of my navel. Brown gunk crusted the skin, which was apparently normal, where "normal" was redefined as "awful."

All this posed more than an aesthetic downer—the stretching process itself tormented me. At night the itchiness made me whimper, then hobble-run to the bathroom for wet, cold towels. I'd swaddle myself, panting with urgency. A few times I gave in to all-out scratching, writhing like Friso when he felt too clean.

This was supposedly normal, too, though Dr. Internet, who took my questions at all hours, thought it might be a rare liver condition that afflicted 0.1 percent of women and mysteriously caused stillbirth. I searched my body for the signature rash of that syndrome, finding none, wearing myself out.

Aside from the skin woes, the Overhang no longer just dangled between my legs. It had swelled laterally, so that even sitting splayed didn't alleviate the sensation of sticky, heavy weight pressed on my thighs. It felt like a damp duffel of Jell-O and doll parts. It dangled close to the top of my genitals, poised for a hostile takeover.

"Yes," Dr. Young said over the phone. "That's called vaginal disappearance. You can never wear pants again, only diapers."

No, of course she did not. "That's normal," she said. "The babies have to go somewhere."

ONE DAY, Ken and I actually cuddled in bed. His skin was warm, hair freshly cut. When he turned to me, his bearded face and brown eyes were so familiar and so missed, I shivered. All other aches and worries vanished into our nearness. I longed for the day I could sleep in bed next to him. Forget cosleeping with two infants—I wanted to cosleep with my man.

A new thought took root along with my stretch marks. *I'm so done with this pregnancy.* At night, with an itchy-stretchy-moody mind, I cruised the chat rooms and baby sites to find out what happened to babies born at thirty-two weeks. It was so much later than thirty-one weeks! I thought I'd heard thirty-two was a milestone. Many women online seemed to think it was A-okay. To my disappointment, thirty-two-week-old twins still toured the NICU, and the pictures weren't much more hopeful than those of babies born at thirty-one.

I did find other mothers-to-be, from the United States and abroad, declaring their doneness with twin pregnancy, and their plans to beg for C-sections at thirty-four weeks. Thus began my own mental bargaining, a silent discussion, mostly monologue, of negotiating the numbers. *I'll carry to thirty-four weeks, but that's it. Okay, fine—thirty-five, but they will be take-home babies!* A friend of mine from grad school had had her babies at thirty-five weeks, I argued to my non-existent opponent, and they were fine. I couldn't make it to thirty-eight weeks, and that was that. It was like what Dr. Abrams had once said: we'd have our babies; the only questions were how and when.

They say bargaining is one of the stages of grief, but it

also applied to agony. It felt like a sliver of power. In the corners of my mind, I still wore the pants.

I TRIED TO KEEP my plans quiet, but they leaked out over breakfast, as I scrambled eggs, Friso crunched kibble, and Ken checked headlines.

"Do you think they'll come early?" I asked.

"We don't know." He had returned to the first-trimester "we," as if to attach jumper cables from his rational machinery to my faltering engine.

"I'm ready for them to be out. Now."

"I know," he said, flapping the newspaper.

"But what do you *think*?"

He gently revved the gas. "We should take it day by day."

If I had a sudden C-section, it could be with any doctor. I hated the idea of a random surgeon, a meet and greet with scalpels in hand, but I managed not to worry about that, as something I couldn't control. Of course, plenty of things I couldn't control still brought worry, like the small earthquakes that rattled our house every other day, jiggling teacups, upsetting Friso.

These seismic tremors hadn't been enough to tip a vase, but the furniture clacked and the walls thundered. Then silence. It was a reminder that even the ground beneath us wasn't stable, could shift any second. How would I get to the hospital for my C-section if the bridge collapsed? What if I got trapped beneath piles of plaster? Didn't the odds of that increase every day that passed?

Any way I sliced it, sooner seemed better. The balanced

part of my brain was being squeezed to smaller quarters, like my bladder.

Since I couldn't sway Ken, I told Tess my plan for the babies to come early.

"I'm sure they'll be fine," she agreed.

I asked our fabulous housekeeper, Patricia, what she thought.

"I feel, four more weeks," she said.

"Me, too!" I gushed. She held her duster. I sprawled on the couch. We smiled and laughed. Together, we'd made this decision.

Now I had to schedule Dr. Young.

"It would be bad if they came now," Dr. Young said.

Pantsless on her table, I hugged two pillows. I'd hiked up the Bellaband, the rest of me still covered beneath my pleated pink shirt, technically a "tunic," and therefore providing coverage for my ass. The top's empire waist fanned out enough to accommodate my huge bump—now officially the size of a forty-week singleton pregnancy. Given the itching, the tunic was the only thing I could stand, and in fact even loved. I'd worn it for days, a gift from my mother, from a special website for women pregnant with multiples.

"Do we have to wait for thirty-eight weeks for the C-section?" I kept my voice calm, as if to nudge her toward the obvious, the way Ken did with me.

"If we do it before thirty-eight weeks, we have to do an amnio to check lung development. That has risks of its own."

"Aren't lungs developed by thirty-four weeks?"

"We always have to check. Believe me, it's better to have them in longer."

I sighed, swallowed a sob. "It's awful."

"You're small. There aren't too many places for the baby to go but out."

"Exactly. I want them out."

She crossed the room, for a speculum. "You'll have all the time in the world to make them pay for this," she said lightly.

She really said that, and I laughed.

I loved her for not talking about miracles, how it would all be worth it, having my whole family at once. Treat crazy with crazy, she'd gambled. It worked.

FOR THE EXAM, I had Ken count backward from 100 by 6.5. It went by in a jiffy, where a jiffy was defined as a unit of time rarely experienced in twin pregnancy. My cervix, like my mind, was firmly closed.

At the end, Dr. Young helped me clarify the fine print of early delivery. "Thirty-two weeks is not the magic number. If you go into labor now, we try to stop it. Thirty-five and onward, we let it go. Thirty-four, we would see. Think of that as your goal."

It seemed impossibly distant. "I'm tired and burnt out. This Overhang is torture, and it's itchy." I curled my fingers in the air over the bump, pantomiming my desire to claw it off.

"Let me look."

Straightening the napkin over my lost privates, I lifted the tunic again. Dr. Young, Ken, and I looked at the bump together, as if observing the model 3-D maps in a visitor center. I reached down and touched the lower hemisphere of deep, heated striations.

"Have you tried using lotion?" Dr. Young asked.

"I slather on kukui oil and expensive maternity crap." I'd given up on coconut.

"You could try something else," she said.

"Do you think it could be choriostastis?" I asked.

"*Cholestasis*. Do your hands and feet itch?"

"No," I admitted.

"It's pretty rare. About one in one thousand. There is a test for it, though."

I wrinkled my nose, shook my head. I would do anything to avoid another intrusion or extraction. On the way home, we bought a bottle of oatmeal lotion, one I'd read about online.

I complained again to Tess by phone.

"Kate Gosselin used to put Vaseline on her bump, and Saran Wrap," she said, referring to the reality-TV star who'd had six kids in one pregnancy, in addition to twins.

"Ew," I said, though by dinner I'd sent Ken back to the store, and by the time we parked by the TV for *Survivor*, I was lubed and wrapped.

"Did I tell Dr. Young about this itch?" I asked.

"I think you made it pretty clear," he said.

On their island, the stranded contestants schemed and wept and battled. Ken rubbed my feet. Friso cuddled behind us. Two small earthquakes shook the house.

Week Thrity-Three:

The Overhang

The Overhang, a sticky basketball between my thighs, itched around the clock. The first sleepless night, I took Benadryl, which left me wired and thirsty. Despite the box's warning of "drowsiness," I spent the small hours hobbling to the bathroom. The next evening, I figured I'd plunge to exhausted sleep, but the mound tingle-burned so much I had to strip down and drape it in towels. Desperate, I ventured out the following day for cotton sheets and organic pajamas, thinking I had an allergy. Instead, the next day's dark period found me bug-eyed beneath brand-new bedding, all my worst thoughts reprised in a symphonic blast. *I made a huge mistake doing IVF. I was happy before, and now it's all shit. I'm so worn out. I feel deformed and ugly and miserable. I'm not cut out for this. I'm too small for twins, in body and spirit.*

This dragged on until we reached Dr. Silverman's, on a chilly morning just before Thanksgiving. The office seemed empty, the staff focused, determined to close early. A woman we hadn't met yet greeted us in the lobby, peeking at my chart. "You're carrying twins," she said. "I have twin boys myself."

I perked up, focused my eyes. A twin mom: someone who could *get it*. Maybe my sister *was* right: everyone had twins. Bird-boned in black leggings, she had kind eyes behind square glasses, her dark hair pulled back. Her name tag read DAWN.

"How was it at thirty-three weeks for you?" I asked.

"I was just leaving the hospital, after five weeks there."

"Oy." At least I got to suffer in the comfort of our home.

"My boys are in high school now." One played lacrosse. The other liked to row.

In the dim maze of the stress-test area, she directed me to bed one, with its rails. Ken, Dawn, and I all faced the machine, and Dawn squeezed the ultrasound condiment onto the tattered skin of my midsection.

"They've moved since last time," she announced during the scan. "They are both transverse, with their heads on the right, feet on the left."

"Is that why I can't lie on my right side?"

"Those heads are like two bowling balls." She just said "heavy," but I got the idea.

"Why can't they be up and down?"

"It's not necessarily better to have them head down," Dawn said. "The weight can be overwhelming." She mimed a woman walking with a grimace, clutching her vagina.

I laughed. "So, this is normal?" I waved my hands over the bump, desperate for that label. I flashed back to the day with Dr. Marion at the fertility clinic, how I'd barely given a thought to her warnings about twin-pregnancy risks. Now, I thought of little else.

"Totally," she said. "Baby B has more fluid, but not a

whole lot more. A much bigger problem is to have not enough. One guy probably pees a lot." She said it in the tone of "boys will be boys."

No one so far had treated this casually. The doctors had their reasons for hedging—not so the techs. With Dawn, I could talk twin mom to twin mom. I let some craziness out of the steam valve of confession. "I can't make it to thirty-eight weeks. I want them out *now*." I told her I had a packed hospital bag in the trunk.

"You never know," she said.

Dawn fiddled with the sensors, placing one hockey puck high, two low. I sighed, torn between my sense of time wasted and my feeling of calm reassurance. The readings flipped in and out on the red digital display, the machine churning out its long page, like a lie-detector test. I already knew it wouldn't be a good reading with the babies in full squirm.

"We can do the bio-profile—I saw all the movements. Ten out of ten for both." She reviewed them with Ken: movement, tone, breathing, fluid, heart rate.

"You should call them 'graceful body movements,'" I added.

No, I actually kept quiet. "Being polite is the lowest energy expenditure," Ken liked to say. I didn't agree. It took tremendous effort to be civil, but I tried to curb my outbursts.

"What about contractions?" I asked.

She studied the third line's bumpy trail. "Yes. No. You have an irritable uterus."

"That's not all," I said.

Dawn laughed. "You'll get your motor back chasing those boys around."

"Someday I'll stop itching, too," I said, sneaking a gripe. "The itching is insane."

"Has anyone tested you for cholestasis?"

"Doc said it's unlikely."

"Let's test you in case. That'll deliver you early."

The nurses led me to a back room, in camaraderie, almost festive. We were hunting down the Complication, the Big One.

Dawn called Dr. Young for authorization, then spent another twenty minutes looking for "the green vials."

"We could wait," I said, knowing everyone wanted to go home and baste turkeys.

"No, let's do it," Dawn insisted.

Green vials appeared. I slumped on a stool, in a space that looked like a supply closet. For once, I didn't mind the pause. I didn't feel afraid, either of the test or of its outcome. I kept thinking of the word "delivery," as in *you will be delivered*. It sounded spiritual, redemptive. That notion kept my breathing slow. The summit was in sight, the oxygen thin. The stakes were impossibly high. I had to keep going.

"Sorry about this," an unknown nurse said, the syringe at my elbow crease.

"It's practically a massage at this point," I told her.

She tied off my arm with a rubber strip and stuck the needle through my skin. I barely felt the poke.

Week Thirty-Four:

The Twin-Pregnancy Terrorist

"Could something be wrong?" I asked one morning, again in the kitchen, as I sprinkled raisins and walnuts on my oatmeal. "I feel almost normal." This despite the Over-hang, which drooped so far down I could only lean, not sit, on the bar-height chair, which I'd angled away from the table. That way, I could reach my bowl around the bump, rather than flapping my too-short dinosaur arms above its mass.

Ken waited by the sighing coffee machine. "You slept last night."

"Except for that fit of scratching," I said.

"And whatever caused all that moaning." Finally, Ken ferried a cup of decaf to my outstretched hands. I shuddered at the first sweet sip. "My arm got pinned, like that guy who got stuck under a boulder for a hundred twenty-seven hours. They made a movie about him."

"Don't say it."

"He had to cut his own arm off. Luckily, mine just went numb." In the faint moonlight, I'd watched my veins swell, incredulous.

Ken embraced my shoulders, our crooked hug. "Four more weeks," he said.

"I used to be agile," I said.

"I know."

"You don't."

"Maybe not."

There was nothing to do but wait—wait for the babies to grow, wait for the days to pass, wait to feel better. I'd repacked the hospital bag, first a small one and later a whole suitcase, with my own pajamas, bathrobe, socks, slippers, and soaps. Time was the boulder bigger than my bump, the one I couldn't budge.

When Ken left for the lab, I decided to get cash, which we'd need no matter what: for the emergency room, the earthquake, or more days at home—they all seemed equally likely. Outside the bank, having hefted myself from the car, I frowned at the three-person line for the ATM, and then, magically, everyone stepped aside. For all the waiting I endured, the waiting in lines had mostly stopped. It felt tremendous, this collective kindness. It hurt to stand, and people let me pass. I murmured my thanks to all but the security guard, who chimed in, as he had weeks earlier, "You're about to pop."

"And you are almost completely bald."

No, I did not say that.

"*Popping* is not my thing," I replied gently—not the greatest comeback, but managed with a smile. That day, I held fear at bay. In the long hours lying still, I'd been drifting back through memory, lingering on anyone I'd ever known to go through an illness.

I thought about a friend from junior high whose mother had been diagnosed with breast cancer at age thirty-eight. From the vantage of thirteen, that had seemed old. She'd crumbled fast. Toward the end, she'd given her daughter a card with undecipherable scribble. My friend had wept, and I'd tried to console, secretly wishing the mother had written something so beautiful, wise, and loving that her leaving would be less sad. Being a mother, and being close to death, meant a soft light should shine. Even on the morning of her last breath, this woman didn't accept that she would die. The words of comfort never came.

While I knew my own suffering was nothing, *nothing*, compared with hers, I felt the presence of death in this making of life, and in that sensation I found not a shred of insight, peace, or enlightenment. Glowing tunnels, grand patterns, and mystical truths did not unfold, forging me a finer self for my sons. Instead, I felt tired and afraid. I couldn't read or rest, much less record clear thoughts. I craved the end and nothing else.

At home, I snuck another quarter cup of decaf. If I watched TV and took a nap, soon enough Ken would be back from work. I told myself that the clock didn't stop, even if I felt itchy and misunderstood. I would be delivered, and the babies would come, whether or not anyone—a guy at the bank, strangers on the street, or even my family—ever *got it* about this twin pregnancy.

The phone rang.

"It's Dr. Young," came the greeting.

I felt special. "What's up?"

"Did you see the *Survivor* finale?" she asked.

No, she did not say that.

She sounded serious. "Your blood tests came back. You do have cholestasis of pregnancy." I'd already forgotten the green-vial blood draw, along with the details of the disease. Dr. Young had numbers. "It's a problem with your liver. The normal range for bile in your system is between eleven and nineteen. Your levels are at sixty-one."

"Oh," I said, knuckling my sternum.

"We're moving your C-section up a few weeks, probably to December fifteenth, and I'd like to start you on medication tonight."

"But my hands and feet aren't itchy. There's no rash," I said, my Internet studies resurfacing like eighth-grade algebra. I'd been longing for an earlier due date, but I felt suddenly queasy and ashamed. *Wait! I changed my mind. This can't be right.*

"It can also be excessive itching that presents without a rash."

I paused. I had that in spades. Longfellow had bloodstains now. Every night I moaned, scratched, and soaked, blaming lotions, polyester, detergent. "Is it dangerous?"

"The reason we do the C-section early is that there are some risks associated with cholestasis. Early labor, mainly. But the big one, and I don't want you to freak out when I say this, is stillbirth."

The word hung in the air, a guillotine above us. *Don't freak out.* I reached down and caressed the bump. *My babies.* "So why wait until thirty-six weeks?"

"All your doctors together came up with that number. It's about balancing prematurity with the risks of the cholestasis. Most of the negative outcomes are when you wait to deliver."

Waiting. It really could be deadly.

"I'm glad you're telling me," I said finally. Her phrase "all your doctors" echoed. I blushed. I was so lucky.

"I wasn't sure if I should, but decided yes."

More quiet on the line.

"I'm trying to stay calm, but I'm scared." The phone in my hand shook, banging against my forehead and jaw.

"The medication will help," Dr. Young said. "Can you give me that pharmacy number again?"

I found the number, my mind unspooling like a ball of yarn. What if I hadn't complained so voraciously to Dawn? I would never have been diagnosed. I had complained so much to Dr. Young about so many things, the itching had gotten lost in the pile. I'd wrinkled my nose at her suggestion to test. Still, without the ongoing complaints, I might have gone to term with the babies marinating in my poison.

On the other hand, what if I had complained less? Could I have avoided this syndrome altogether? Might I have made this toxic bile by dint of my toxic speech, the body's mirror of the mind's activity? Couldn't I have been more stoic? Probably not, I realized.

I felt reluctant to let Dr. Young off the line. No one could die with the doctor on the line, right? If I hung up, I'd be alone with the word "stillbirth."

"Don't go poking around the Internet," Dr. Young said.

"Okay," I lied.

We said our goodbyes. I'd see her the next day.

AT THE END OF THAT AFTERNOON, Ken plunked down at the head of the table while I stared at my hands, still shaking.

"Dr. Young called. I have that thing they tested me for, cholestasis." I wanted to put a good spin on it. "It's pretty amazing that it was the techs who did the test—none of the doctors did."

"What does it mean?" he asked.

I told him about the buildup of bile, how we would move the C-section. The guilt of that loomed like the first big storm of a season, the one that stirred the leaves and silenced the birds, the one where you looked out at the gray sky and realized you weren't at all prepared. I made myself keep talking. "The thing is . . . they do the C-section early because . . . there's a chance of stillbirth."

Ken was silent.

I decided I wouldn't say the s-word again, ever.

I'd cried throughout the pregnancy, but the tears that came now were different. Someone told me once that with real sadness, tears were colder, and salty, and the stream on my face had the ocean's bitter ice.

Ken came over for another sideways hug, so different than the morning's. "It's okay," he said softly, without conviction.

"I want them. I want them both. I've been complaining so much about twins, and giving birth early, but I want them." It felt like the day Dr. Marion had put them inside me, multiplied by every second that had since passed. Nothing so far matched my urge to protect those two lives.

"I've been complaining so much," I whispered. "I mean, what if . . . after all this?"

"Listen. We are a team. You and me. I have it on my chalkboard at work, K plus K equals Team Goldberg. It's a rule of physics. Whatever happens, we'll get through it together."

Ken stayed solid. I had to do the same. I pulled myself together. Getting hysterical wouldn't help anyone, even though I felt myself to blame, for the tainted bath in my body, and for wishing the birth sooner. I'd suffered so much over the doctors, the tests, the pain, the expense, all the while getting reports of healthy babies.

The boys flailed, and I rubbed their feisty limbs and prayed. *Keep kicking.* Ken left to Pharmaca to get the Actigall, pills that translated my panic to the runs and nausea all night long. I padded back and forth to the bathroom, trying to be blank and to bear the terrible weight.

At the window, watching shadows in our wintry yard, I knew something I hadn't through this whole twin pregnancy: I was the one who didn't *get it*. Not my doctors, not my father, not my mother, not Ken. They got it. I was the one who missed it. This wasn't a bump, an Overhang, a boulder. It was our *sons*. They were stuck inside me, until the doctor cut them out.

WEEK THIRTY-FIVE:

Deliverance

I f you have to take Actigall, you might as well chase it with bad beer and tainted beans, because you will be rushing to the bathroom every hour anyway. Though the itching stilled, once again I couldn't sleep at night, for the constant trips to the toilet. I dutifully took each pill, twice a day. I followed every medical instruction, even stuff that seemed silly, like "kick counts" for each baby. I forced eggs, chicken, rice, broccoli, and spinach down my gullet, swallowed my vitamins and Zantac, parked myself for bed rest at four o'clock each day.

The pharmacy sheet for Actigall said, *Call your doctor if the symptoms get worse*, so I did that, too. On a Saturday, I figured my chances of chatting with an MD were equal to getting Michelle Obama's direct line to discuss her garden, but I called Dr. Young's office anyway.

The medical assistant actually laughed when I said I wanted to speak to a doctor, then took my name, birth date, due date, and Social Security number. "You can ask me your question," she said, having verified my existence.

I described my ballistic bowels.

She paused. "Um. Ummmmm."

It lasted so long, I tried rephrasing. "I'll take the Actigall if I have to, but I'm worried about dehydration."

"Ummmmmmmmm."

I waited, confidence waning.

Finally she spoke. "Don't mix the Actigall with Zantac or prenatal vitamins," she suggested. "Take each set at the same time every day." This would have involved bi-hourly pill routines, nearly impossible to track.

After more *ummmm*ing, through which I heard keys typing, she finally burst out with another answer. "Take the Actigall. There's no other medicine. We'll find another med to stop the diarrhea."

Two hours later, a Dr. Lee called me back. I felt excited he had a medical degree, though he seemed to be watching football while we talked, because halfway through the conversation, he'd be surprised by something we'd covered earlier.

"Wait, you have diarrhea?"

"That's mostly why I called."

In the end he said he'd call someone at Dr. Silverman's. They must have had a doctor-to-doctor hotline. I felt relieved, until he asked, "What's the drug, again?"

A few hours later, Dr. Lee called back after he'd spoken to a Dr. Stone. "The drug doesn't actually help with cholestasis. It's only to stop the itching."

Bottle in hand, I lowered my forehead to the table.

IN THE FARTHEST-BACK ROOM of Dr. Young's, in the weak light from the high, skinny window, Ken helped hoist me onto the table, where I immediately peeled off my pants and underwear, shedding down to my pink twin tunic. I kicked the rest onto a chair. "Can you cover the underwear?"

"Wow, what's going on?" Ken asked.

"I'm compliant now." I'd bargain with the gods, and the doctors, too. I would be stoic, no matter that my butt felt crushed like an old pillow and my legs splayed at a crazy angle around the bump. *Please let the boys be okay.*

After twenty minutes of waiting, my eyes sprang a leak.

Ken handed me a tissue.

"I'm like that stupid broken clock," I said, nodding toward the frozen timepiece on the wall. "I feel so stuck."

Ken reached up, took it down. He set the hands to 9:20. "There," he said. "It's perfect now," and replaced it on the hook.

Galvanized by the pause in my tears, he darted his eyes around the room, in search of a further distraction. "Look at the bright side—do you want some free medical supplies?" He gestured at the swabs and clamps on a metal table.

"You're going to get in trouble," I said, but a faint chuckle pushed through.

"How about some Q-tips?" He grabbed a fistful. "I bet these would be good for cleaning bottles."

"They're going to see you!" I whispered.

"Or maybe I could do the ultrasound." He approached the machine. "I'd be good at it by now." He tapped the keys. "Let's invent a patient. Friso Goldberg."

I blew my nose, shaking my head.

Ken took out his camera. "Now smile and look tranquil."

I raised a middle finger—though not at him. "How about a salute?"

"Get rid of the tissue, and straighten that finger!"

The lens snapped four times, and in the last frame, I accidentally smiled for real, so that when Dr. Young came in at 9:30 a.m., she mistakenly thought I was normal and fine. I hoped she would give me magic information about cholestasis, to take the edge off my fear. *Let the boys be okay.*

We exchanged hellos, and she gave me a printout about cholestasis from the American Pregnancy Association. "Did you look at the Internet?"

"I did," I confessed. "I know it's better for babies to bake longer, but is it safe?"

"We have all talked, and thirty-six weeks seems like the best choice." Dr. Young sounded firm.

Time stopped like the clock on the wall. I had to choose. Could I trust my doctors? Could I trust anyone? The babies? My body? God? I trusted Ken, that much I knew, and he trusted that long, uncertain list. Maybe, just maybe, I could, too. Having whimsically decided to put two embryos inside me almost eight months earlier, I now made my second life-altering, pants-off decision. Right there, butt on vinyl, I decided I could have faith. It wasn't a flood. It was more like opening the front door to a familiar stranger from whom I wished an endless favor.

Dr. Young kept talking. "Before the C-section, no food or drink after two a.m. Surgery at ten a.m. sharp." We couldn't start late, she said. "I have an appointment that afternoon."

"Christmas play?" I ventured.

Dr. Young smiled. "As a matter of fact, yes. My daughter's."

I nodded, pleased. She wouldn't plan to go to *The Nut-cracker* if she thought we were going to die, right? I felt reluctant to leave the office. Here, I could be whisked to the hospital. Once I got home, I'd be stranded like a poached manatee in the daybed in the nursery.

"Maybe the night before we should stay in a hotel nearby," I said, worried about Bay Bridge traffic.

"There's a Ritz right up the road," Dr. Young said. "Doctor's orders."

She didn't say "doctor's orders," but she did mention the Ritz, which was how we found ourselves, at the end of week thirty-five, at a swanky hotel only an hour from home. It was the fanciest place we'd ever stayed—as far from normal as I felt, and a five-minute drive to the hospital. This way, Dr. Young wouldn't leave me with a stranger to go see her kid as a sugarplum because my surgical spot had ticked by while a gun-waving nut clogged cars on the bridge. My fresh and fragile faith did not extend to highways, tolls, and tunnels.

At the end of the week, parked in the Ritz's half-moon driveway, Ken unwedged me from the shotgun seat into a waiting wheelchair. I wore my trusty pink polyester twin tunic. I itched everywhere, feeling lightheaded, achy, and giddy, as I watched Ken unload the trunk. I checked my phone: pictures of Friso from Tess; texts from Linda; e-mails from my sister, mom, and dad, all wishing luck. I felt their support as clearly as I felt the two babies inside me. The presence of death, that cold shadow of possibility at the edge of a birth, also brought with it knowledge of love.

A guy in uniform gathered our suitcases while Ken wheeled me into the lushly carpeted lobby. I didn't wear my glasses, since mild blindness helped me to detach, but I could tell the blur of lit Christmas trees and crystal chandeliers gave the place a lovely glow. I moaned with my head lolled back. Four legs kicked my pelvis and my ribs, and I softly touched those feet and fists.

"I'm giving birth tomorrow," I told the two women at the check-in desk. "Twins. By C-section."

They oohed and aahed, peering down at the bulk of me —of us. I'd tipped sideways a bit in the wheelchair, the bump lopsided, almost moving without me.

"We're going to upgrade you to a junior suite."

They really said this.

They handed us two card keys and sent us off with white terry-cloth baby bibs that read RITZ-CARLTON, SAN FRANCISCO.

"These are going to look great covered in spit-up," Ken said.

"I wish they'd added an adult bib for me."

As he rolled me to the elevator, it struck me that several pregnancy fantasies were converging at the last minute—the plush surroundings, the room service, the upgrade. I felt appreciation for it all, and a singular focus of longing. *Let the boys be okay.*

On our floor, Ken pushed my chair forward, back, forward, back, rolling while I laughed, which hurt, though I didn't want to stop. In the room, they brought us chocolate-covered strawberries. We would spend our last childless night in luxury. In the morning, we would check into even more expensive digs, the priciest place you can stay in America: the hospital.

Week Thrity-Six:

The Baby Library

Throughout my twin pregnancy, I'd given surprisingly little thought to the birth. "C-section" sounded more like the midbalcony area of a theater than front-row seating at my own surgery. One of the perks was not having to ponder or prepare—no videos, no Lamaze, no debate about drugs. I would be heavily medicated. For months, everyone who'd ever had one had reassured me it was not a big deal.

I'd recently called Tina to confirm.

"It was a little gnarly," she had admitted. "It was weird being awake."

"You can't feel from the waist down, though, right?"

"Well . . ."

I didn't want to know more. "But you bounced back quickly, didn't you?"

"I felt much better after six weeks."

"Six weeks!"

"*Now* the stories come," I sulked to Ken later.

"You hate people scaring you," he reminded me.

"I guess that's true." I appreciated the restraint of my C-section sisters.

Now the day had arrived, and as the minutes ticked, I still didn't think about spinals or scalpels or the *s*-word. I focused on the fact that within hours, with the help of surgeons, Starbucks, and God, we'd finally meet our sons.

I mention Starbucks because when Dr. Young and Dr. Abrams greeted us in preop, each held a green-and-white paper cup. They seemed relaxed, in contrast with the tension of the room, that final container of waiting. The bland white cube, with washable surfaces and glass walls, gave the impression the place could be locked down, hosed down, or both. We chatted about our night at the Ritz, as if the four of us were upscale tourists, as if I weren't filled with poison bile, as if I weren't tumbling out of the bottom of my twin tunic. Then another massively pregnant woman appeared.

"Twin mom walking," Dr. Abrams said.

No, he said only, "Here's another twin mom."

Like me, she bulged precipitously, despite her height. At one elbow was a man who must have been her husband, and at the other, a woman I decided was her sister, her next in command.

"Good luck," I said.

She offered a wan smile, her face drained of color. I'd turned pale, too, almost gray, in the last week, from anemia and fear. I felt stretched beyond all limits.

After that, things moved either slow or fast—the trip to the OR, Ken in a blue gown and puffy cap, tubes in my arms and between my legs. They did the spinal, an event that under other circumstances would have horrified me. Instead I thought, *It's almost done.* In those last moments, I finally grasped the temporary nature of the pregnancy.

I surrendered my body. I knew all the critiques of modern medical birth: the lost art of midwifery, the unnecessary rise of C-sections, the women stripped of the sacred. I had heard people grieved when they weren't allowed to labor. For me, twin gestation was labor enough. Anything that delivered my boys safely was holy in my eyes.

Ken readied our iPod with shaky hands. The doctors donned their masks. They seemed both surprised and pleased at our island ukulele selection.

"We're going to Hawaii," Dr. Abrams laughed. "Great."

As they had warned us they would, Dr. Young and Dr. Abrams conversed from the incision onward, like gregarious sushi chefs beyond the counter—or, in this case, a curtain. I never heard their words. Intense movement rocked my abdomen—not pain, but a sensation too strange to name, a pulling in the core.

"Some women push for twelve hours," Dr. Abrams said to me when a noise escaped my throat. "You're going to be uncomfortable for another twenty minutes."

Aside from the disturbing fact of talking to my surgeon during surgery, this comforted me. The anesthesiologist had her face to my ear, and Ken kept his eyes locked on mine. They both held my hands. *It's almost over,* I kept thinking. *Almost done.*

As they reached for Baby A from the Overhang, I groaned, not so much in agony as in shock, an earthquake rocking my organs, the Big One. I felt outside myself, and also stuck. The room turned to fragments: bloody latex gloves; fluorescent light tubes; remote, garbled talk.

An infant cried.

"We're going for the second one!" Dr. Abrams shouted.

"You are doing so awesome," Ken said to me, hoarse.

A second infant cried.

You're born alone and you die alone, the saying goes, but my twins were born together, in a crowded room, just as they'd been conceived. A team of waiting protectors surrounded them—two surgeons, three nurses, an anesthesiologist, Ken, and, of course, me—exhausted, thrilled, scared, and ready, as much as I could be. I cried, too, elated.

Someone placed the babies high in my arms. I turned my head, touching their foreheads with mine.

"They are five pounds, six ounces, and five pounds, thirteen," Ken whispered.

I felt stunned, speechless. The world went light. I greeted my sons and kissed my husband, and then, mercifully, the doctors knocked me out.

I SANK IN AND OUT of consciousness. Women in scrubs shoveled me from the stretcher to a bed with a flat board. As they scooted me center-cot, my limbs thwumped, as if detached, lost to morphine. For months, I hadn't been able to escape my body. Now, I barely felt it. Ken stood by, grasping my hand, asking over and over, "How are you?"

"Fine," I said, surprised at the rubbery thickness of my lips. "How are the boys?"

"Healthy and whole."

"Tell me the weights again?" I slurred.

"Five pounds, six ounces, and five pounds, thirteen."

"That's good, right?"

"That's great. No NICU. They're perfect."

The nurses seemed talkative and energetic as they reinserted a needle in the arm—my arm, apparently—then topped off the plastic bag that dangled from a pole. *Keep it coming, girls.* My legs were bundled in thick, air-filled "floaties" that pulsed up and down, breathing like Darth Vader. These compression pants were like the birth itself: not awful but weird, like Tina had said, uncomfortable, and also reassuring. Inside the pants, a roller hummed up and down from thigh to ankle, though one kept jamming below the knee. Several times, we called the nurse, who jangled it back into motion.

I floated in a bubble of awe, relief, and morphine. At the edges of this new island called motherhood, postpartum waves crashed on the shore, faint but audible. Then, in the middle of the first night, a beeping sound blared, like a miniature dump truck driving in reverse. The trousers had shut off.

I woke Ken in the dark room. As San Francisco twinkled beyond the window, it took me a moment to grasp where I was. "My pants died!"

"I'll call the nurse again."

"Babies okay?" The pants weren't an omen, but I asked from habit, even while drugged, about anything in sets.

"They're in the Baby Library." That's what we called the ward's twenty-four-hour nursery. Ken had been ferrying the boys back and forth, showing his wristband for entry and for "checkout," for feeding, holding, marveling.

"Should we get them?"

"It's two a.m. Let them rest," he said. "You rest, too."

I secretly felt relieved, which made me afraid. What if I never felt awake? How would I care for two preemies in this condition? Even through the morphine haze, this thought sounded a siren of alarm, alongside the beep of the busted pants.

Numbing liquid dripped to my arm. A catheter cord ran from my bladder. Once, this would have upset me, my body hooked to multiple machines. Now, I wanted only sleep. Finally, the nurse jumped the leg-hugging rafts and I sailed back out on the cool white noise.

THE SECOND DAY IN THE HOSPITAL, as morning fog shrouded the city outside, an insanely chipper nurse said, "Time to stop morphine."

"It's working well," I said, my tongue like wool.

"We always change after a day."

"I won't get addicted," I insisted, a newly minted narco-mommy.

Both nurses gave a hearty laugh, as did Ken.

"I won't," I said, indignant. "What's funny?"

"We'll get you on the aspirin," they said.

Actually, they said "Toradol," which sounded like a turtle tranquilizer, whereas I wanted elephant meds. With the puffed pants tight around my still-swelling legs, with my midsection ever expanding, I didn't feel keen to experience my body. Despite my protest, they took away my precious opiates, and then the wheezing pants.

A few hours later, I could speak coherently again. My mind cleared of mist, enough for me to be pleased when the nurses transferred us to a bigger room, one they saved for twins.

"I'll go check the boys out of the Baby Library," Ken said, having settled our suitcases and plugged in all our phones, tablets, and laptops.

I needed a plug for myself, a reboot, a software update. I felt stranded between screens, with the spinning beach ball. Giving birth to twins didn't mean I could parent them. I couldn't even walk to the bathroom on my own, could barely turn over in the metal-sided bed. My midsection had grown even larger with postsurgical fluid but felt distressingly unstable, as if my organs had been ransacked, maybe even sold.

Ken returned with the babies in wheeled, cradle-size cots with plastic sides. Meanwhile, I could barely sit up, the muscles of my stomach no longer responsive, so Ken propped me upright, then placed a baby in each arm, atop the aching midsection.

I couldn't stop staring. One boy had a round face, puffy cheeks, and a berry mouth. "That's Max," I said. His brother had huge eyes and wrinkled skin. "This is Sam."

"That's what I think, too," Ken said. We'd had the names for years, but it took only seconds to see who they were.

I held Sam and Max, two tiny packets tucked in flannel, with blue-and-pink hats on their dainty heads. I hugged their bodies, stared at their mouths and eyes and hands and feet. No one had told me how beautiful this would feel.

Actually, almost everyone had. Now I believed.

Still, I felt relieved to hand them back, blind with worry, crushed with fatigue.

DR. ABRAMS AND DR. YOUNG came in separate visits to check bandages and exclaim their delight. "You were all baby," Dr. Abrams said. "We were talking in the surgery about the insanity of having twins on your frame."

"So it *was* extreme," I said, as if I needed a doctor to confirm. They could say that now, while so much more went unsaid: the years that had passed, the doubt, struggle, and faith.

"You've got two beautiful boys."

I nodded, wordless with gratitude. I loved those boys, down in the Baby Library.

"Are you walking?" Dr. Abrams asked.

"To the bathroom," I said.

"Maybe try a bit farther."

Within an hour, clinging to a wall rail, I dragged myself into the hall.

My legs felt stiff, each step leaden. I spotted a few other women in robes, some who carried a baby in arms, others who strolled with baby in cart. These mothers appeared shrunken—natural-birth moms, I guessed. Singleton moms. They did not seem to mourn their lack of C-section and swelling, of having been robbed of the complete medical experience. One woman wore actual jeans.

I tried not to compare myself. I heaved one enormous foot forward, and then the other, until something felt awry in my nethers. Back in the bathroom attached to our room, I found I'd bloodied the hospital-issue underwear, the gargantuan, burlap-textured knickers. Luckily, they were disposable, and I flung them into the bin.

In the parallel world in which IVF hadn't worked, we would have been in Tahiti, wedged into a mountainside. It sounded like an impossible heaven of beach, breeze, and ocean, and yet I knew if we'd been there, we'd be longing for this—hospital, birth, babies. Here's something I learned about giving birth to twins: waiting ends, and it's possible to feel devastated, afraid, and, at the same time, insanely content. In this world, we had Max and Sam.

INSTEAD OF VENTURING OUT AGAIN, I took a shower, tilted awkwardly on the bench and holding the removable nozzle. Despite the massiveness and pain, I felt gentle toward my body. It had done amazing work, and I wouldn't look at it with a critical eye. Or any eye. I kept myself covered, even while bathing, with a big washcloth. My center felt disrupted and haphazard, like a burrito that had been emptied and thrown back together.

It took twenty minutes to put on a fresh pair of the hospital underwear. In the journey of pants—from jeans to yoga pants to maternity leggings to skirt pants to compression pants to no pants—these represented the least-sexy way station, a complete crossing-over. I felt safe in them for now, the way they went up over the incision, protective of the line where the babies had come, this wounded flesh. I had imagined this would be tidier, and I realized I'd thought the same about the transition to mothering. All of it, I could now see, turned out to be primitive and messy.

When I was dressed again, exhausted and crampy, Ken helped hoist me back into bed, then left to borrow the babies himself. I drifted in and out of a nap, while nearby he snapped photos of our infant boys. I held them for a while, then fell back to sleep.

The next day, I loaded the hospital jumbo undies with extra pads, in their traditional use, and also as extra cushioning at the incision. I had Ken help me with the ACE bandage/girdle, a four-foot elastic strip that sealed with Velcro, even though I didn't want him to see the post-birth zone. I put on a second pair of underwear, now fully wrapped.

"I should be a Victoria's Secret Angel," I told him.

He laughed. "You're pretty funny."

"I need me some wings."

"You need this." Ken handed me my mobster robe for the trek to the Baby Library. I set out again, still wobbly and slow, but less stiff. My ankles had blown up to dense trapezoids, but I could lift my feet an inch off the floor. Hand on the rail, holding not grasping, I didn't stop this time. At the nursery door, covered in paper Christmas decorations, a woman in white blocked my passage.

"I'm here for Max and Sam," I said, thrusting my band out for her to check. I stared at it myself, the boldest part of its label: MOTHER. It may have been that moment when it finally clicked. I couldn't wait another minute. I peered over her shoulder into the room, scanning the line of carts.

"You have the twins," the nurse said.

"Yeah," I said, with a thousand watts of pride.

She let me pass. Like me, she believed in my tag: MOTHER. I wanted to run inside, but I plowed on in my shuffle. This was how I'd learn to care for two babies— slowly, with terror, tenderness, and determination. Inside, more nurses bustled around me with files and bottles and blankets, flowing past me like I was a rock in a river. No one cared that I wore a gown and girdle, my wounds and looseness bound up and sloppy. I didn't care myself.

Two dozen babies slept in their carts, in a long, ragged row. I found Sam and Max, their beds pushed together, all four eyes closed. The sight of them, side by side, reminded me something I'd known for a while but never let myself say. They had chosen to come together. They had chosen us. They had chosen me. They didn't care that I was flawed, not yet, anyway. They had looked down and seen our house, with its puppy and salt and pepper shakers and rec room and hope, and they'd chosen. I'd chosen them, too.

I asked a nurse to settle them in one cart, which she did. As we walked, I glanced at the other hatted infants down the line, singletons, and all I could think was, *Just one? Where's the other child?* I turned back to my sons. I chose them again, both, together. I rolled Max and Sam from the Baby Library, on permanent loan, this swaddled pair. The hold had been lifted, the wait finally over. I pushed them toward the hall, toward Ken, toward home, dazed at the grace I'd been granted in twins.

Acknowledgments

Thank you to the many beloved people who have cheered me on over the years and who believed in this book: Tina Hartell, Tess Reiche-Johnson, Linda Peckham, Elizabeth MacKenzie, Theo Pauline Nestor, and Lisa Catherine Harper. Thank you to Michelle Hamilton, for reading an early draft, and for always listening, and to Gisele Rainer, for having my back. I send huge thanks to dazzling moms Lynn Wu, Christine Nygaard, and Meredith Samp, and to all the women of Twins by the Bay. These friendships are a blessing beyond compare.

I could not have completed this book without Farm Saefong, who brought so much peace, wisdom, and love to our home. Thank you, Sharon Donovan, awesome agent and bighearted person, for your faith in this project and for sitting next to me at Book Passage. Thank you to Brooke Warner, Annie Tucker, Cait Levin and the rest of the amazing women of She Writes Press. I'm lucky to be in your excellent hands. Thank you to Kelli Uhrich, Sara Chambers, and Crystal Patriarche of SparkPoint Studio. I'm thrilled you're on my team.

Thank you to Leslie Kefauver, reader, editor, extraordinary mom, and dream grandma. Mom, I wouldn't be a writer without your passion, intelligence, and unwavering support. Thank you to Brenda and James Kefauver. Dad, your unflagging enthusiasm for my words means the world. Thank you to Sandra Goldberg and the much-missed Joseph

Goldberg—your love is with me daily. Thank you to Karen Kefauver, social media guru, energetic aunt, and "queen's advisor" on this venture. Thank you to Friso, for keeping my feet warm.

Thank you to the beautiful Samuel and Maxwell, for being yourselves and lighting up my days. Every moment of struggle was worth it to get to you. Above all, thank you, Kenneth Goldberg, father of my children, love of my life. There are no words, yet you always seem to know.

A Brief Glossary of Terms

Bio-profile: fetal biophysical profile

C-section: cesarean section

CVS: chorionic villus sampling

FSH: follicle-stimulating hormone

HSG: hysterosalpingogram

IUI: intrauterine insemination

IVF: in vitro fertilization

MRI: magnetic resonance imaging

Saline sonogram: saline infusion sonohysterography

ABOUT THE AUTHOR

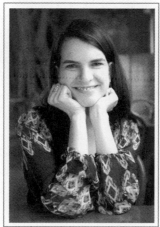

Photo credit: Kenneth Goldberg

MacDowell Fellow and MFA graduate K.K. Goldberg's writing has appeared in the *New York Times* and in numerous literary journals and anthologies, including the *Sun*, the *Gettysburg Review*, the *Alaska Quarterly Review*, the *Chicago Quarterly Review*, and *Best Women's Travel Writing 2009*. A native of Bethesda, Maryland, Kathryn lives in Berkeley with her husband, twin toddlers, and a mischievous bichon.

SELECTED TITLES FROM SHE WRITES PRESS

She Writes Press is an independent publishing company
founded to serve women writers everywhere.
Visit us at www.shewritespress.com.

A Leg to Stand On: An Amputee's Walk into Motherhood by Colleen
Haggerty. $16.95, 978-1-63152-923-8. Haggerty's candid story of how
she overcame the pain of losing a leg at seventeen—and of
terminating two pregnancies as a young woman—and went on to
become a mother, despite her fears.

Make a Wish for Me: A Mother's Memoir by LeeAndra Chergey.
$16.95, 978-1-63152-828-6. A life-changing diagnosis teaches a family
that where's there is love there is hope—and that being "normal" is
not nearly as important as providing your child with a life full of
joy, love, and acceptance.

*Mothering Through the Darkness: Women Open Up About the
Postpartum Experience* edited by Stephanie Sprenger and Jessica
Smock. $16.95, 978-1-63152-804-0. A collection of thirty powerful
essays aimed at spreading awareness and dispelling myths about
postpartum depression and perinatal mood disorders.

Breathe: A Memoir of Motherhood, Grief, and Family Conflict by Kelly
Kittel. $16.95, 978-1-938314-78-0. A mother's heartbreaking account
of losing two sons in the span of nine months—and learning,
despite all the obstacles in her way, to find joy in life again.

Americashire: A Field Guide to a Marriage by Jennifer Richardson.
$15.95, 978-1-938314-30-8. A couple's decision about whether or not
to have a child plays out against the backdrop of their new home in
the English countryside.

Three Minus One: Parents' Stories of Love & Loss edited by Sean
Hanish and Brooke Warner. $17.95, 978-1-938314-80-3. A collection
of stories and artwork by parents who have suffered child loss that
offers insight into this unique and devastating experience.